Opportunities for and barriers to good nutritional health in women of childbearing age, pregnant women, infants under 1 and children aged 1 to 5

Opportunities for and barriers to good nutritional health in women of childbearing age, pregnant women, infants under 1 and children aged 1 to 5

Margaret Reid
Helen Adamson
Department of Public Health
University of Glasgow
2 Lilybank Gardens
Glasgow G12 8RZ

Opportunities for and barriers to good nutritional health

Series co-ordinator and editor
Dr Elizabeth Murphy
School of Social Studies
University of Nottingham

Also available in this series:
Opportunities for and barriers to good nutritional health in minority ethnic groups
Opportunities for and barriers to change in the dietary behaviour of elderly people

This series of reports complements a series of systematic effectiveness reviews also published by the HEA:
Health promotion in older people for the prevention of coronary heart disease and stroke
Health promotion in childhood and young adolescence for the prevention of unintentional injuries
Effectiveness of video for health education
Effectiveness of mental health promotion interventions
Health promotion with young people for the prevention of substance misuse
Health promotion interventions to promote healthy eating in the general population
Effectiveness of oral health promotion
Effectiveness of interventions to promote healthy feeding of infants under one year: a review
Effectiveness of interventions to promote healthy eating in preschool children aged 1–5 years: a review
Effectiveness of interventions to promote healthier living in people from minority ethnic groups: a review
Effectiveness of interventions to promote healthy eating in elderly people living in the community: a review

Forthcoming topics:
Health promotion interventions in the workplace: a review

This work received funding from the Department of Health: the views expressed in this publication are those of the authors and not necessarily those of the Department of Health.

ISBN 0 7521 1156 6

Health Education Authority
Trevelyan House
30 Great Peter Street
London SW1P 2HW

Cover design by Maria Grasso
Printed in Great Britain

Contents

Foreword

This report is one of a series of linked literature reviews, commissioned by the Department of Health, as part of its commitment to protect, promote and improve the nutritional health of the nation. The aim of the series as a whole is to bring together current knowledge about cultural, behavioural, material and societal opportunities for, and barriers to, good nutritional health, so as to inform the development and implementation of interventions which are intended to encourage healthy eating in particular target groups.

This review is concerned with factors which promote healthy eating among women of childbearing age and those who are pregnant, infants under 1 year and children aged between 1 and 5 years. Other target groups covered in this series are:

- ethnic minority groups living in Great Britain
- elderly people.

There is, of course, some common ground between these reviews. For example, the review of ethnic minority groups covers the entire life cycle of the groups under study. It therefore overlaps, to some extent, with the material on pregnant women, women of childbearing age, infants and children up to 5 years who are the focus of this review. No attempt has been made to avoid overlaps and, to that extent, each of the reviews can be considered to be free-standing.

All the reviewers in this series were charged with offering pointers to new ways of formulating and delivering interventions to improve the nutritional health of target groups. Within this overall brief, they were each given the following tasks, in relation to their particular target group:

- to inform policymakers and others of what is already known about opportunities for, and barriers to, good nutritional health
- to offer suggestions on possible interventions which might be expected to overcome identified barriers or take advantage of identified opportunities, which could then be tested in further research
- to inform the design of future dietary intervention strategies to improve their effectiveness
- to identify needs for further research and appropriate research questions.

In parallel with this series of reviews of opportunities for, and barriers to, healthy eating, the Department of Health also commissioned a second set of literature reviews which focus upon the effectiveness of interventions to promote healthier eating, in the same target groups. This parallel set of reviews commissioned through the Health Education Authority in their series, Health promotion effectiveness reviews, focuses explicitly upon the methods, outcomes and effectiveness of existing interventions. Our own series deals with interventions only in so far as they throw light upon the barriers to, or opportunities for, dietary change which are our primary focus. As a result, the two sets of reviews are complementary to one another.

All of these reviews are concerned with factors which influence the dietary behaviours of the healthy population, rather than with the treatment or care of those who are ill. The focus is upon factors which either facilitate or obstruct healthy eating among members of each target group. All the reviewers have taken as their starting point the current best advice on diet and nutrition for the whole population, which is embodied in COMA reports (Department of Health and Social Security, 1988; Department of Health, 1991, 1992a, 1994a, 1994b, 1997). They have been concerned to identify ways in which the nutrition targets set out in the *Health of the nation* White Paper (Department of Health, 1992b) may be met. These targets are summarised in Figure 1.

Saturated fat
To reduce the average percentage of food energy derived by the population from saturated fatty acids by at least 35% by 2005 (from 17% in 1990 to no more than 11%).

Total fat
To reduce the average percentage of food energy derived by the population from total fat by at least 12% by 2005 (from about 40% in 1990 to no more than 35%).

Fig. 1. **Relevant Health of the Nation targets (Department of Health, 1992b)**

- Eating lots of *bread, other cereals and potatoes* and choosing wholemeal, wholegrain or high fibre versions where possible. Avoiding, where possible, fried versions, adding too much fat or rich sauces and dressings.
- Eating lots of *fruit and vegetables* and choosing a wide variety. Avoiding, where possible, adding fat or rich sauces to vegetables and sugar to fruit.
- Eating or drinking moderate amounts of *milk and dairy foods* and choosing lower fat versions where possible.
- Eating moderate amounts of *meat, fish and alternatives* and choosing lower fat versions where possible.
- Eating foods containing *fat* sparingly, choosing *low fat alternatives* and eating *foods containing sugar* not too often.

Fig. 2. **Means by which 'healthy eating' may be achieved**

Food group	Foods	Recommended behaviour for healthy eating
Bread, other cereals and potatoes	Bread and rolls	Eat lots and choose wholemeal, wholegrain, brown or high fibre versions where possible. Avoid adding too much butter, margarine or low fat spread.
	Breakfast cereals	Eat lots and choose high fibre types where possible.
	Pasta, rice and other grains	Eat lots, try brown where possible and avoid adding rich sauces and dressings.
	Potatoes	Eat lots, with the skin on if possible and avoid having them fried too often or served with fat spread.
Fruit and vegetables	Fruit	Eat lots, include a variety and avoid adding sugar or syrupy dressings.
	Vegetables	Eat lots, include a variety and avoid adding butter, margarine, fat spread or rich sauces.
	Salad vegetables	Eat lots, include a variety and avoid mayonnaise and oily dressings where possible.
Milk and dairy products	Milk	Drink moderate amounts and choose semi-skimmed or skimmed where possible.
	Cheese	Eat moderate amounts and choose lower fat cheeses such as Edam, half-fat Cheddar or Camembert.
	Yoghurt and fromage frais	Eat moderate amounts and choose low fat (0.1%) rather than whole milk products.
Meat, fish and alternatives	Meat (includes carcass meat and meat products)	Eat moderate amounts of lean meat with the fat cut off, and cook without added fat and limit the amount and frequency of eating high fat meat products such as pies and pasties.
	Poultry	Eat moderate amounts, without the skin and cook without added fat.
	Fish	Eat moderate amounts, without added fat or batter and eat oily fish twice weekly.
	Eggs	Eat moderate amounts and avoid frying or adding fat where possible.
	Beans	Eat moderate amounts as a naturally low fat alternative to meat.
Foods containing fat Foods containing sugar	Spreading fats: butter, margarine, reduced fat spread	Can be eaten daily, but in very small amounts. Choose low fat alternatives.
	Cooking oils	Can be eaten daily, but in small amounts.
	Mayonnaise and oil-based salad dressings	Can be used daily but in very small amounts. Choose low fat alternatives.
	Cakes, biscuits, pastries, confectionery, crisps, cream, soft drinks	Limit amount and frequency of eating and choose lower fat alternatives. If foods and drinks contain sugar, limit to mealtimes.

***Fig. 3.* Healthy eating behaviours**

Based on guidance provided by the Health Education Authority, Department of Health and MAFF in: *The balance of good health: information for educators and communicators* (Health Education Authority, 1995).

For the purposes of these reviews, 'healthy eating' is defined as eating behaviours which are compatible with achieving the dietary reference values (Department of Health, 1991), which meet these Health of the Nation targets (Department of Health, 1992b). Such 'healthy eating' involves eating the foods from the five food groups in the proportions set out in *The balance of good health* (Health Education Authority, 1995) and summarised in Figure 2.

The eating behaviours which are compatible with healthy eating include, but are not restricted to, those listed in Figure 3. Nutritional issues which are specific to the target groups considered here are discussed in Chapter 1 of this report.

Elizabeth Murphy
Series Co-ordinator and Editor
School of Social Studies
University of Nottingham

References

Department of Health and Social Security (1988). *Present day practice in infant feeding: third report*. Report on Health and Social Subjects No. 32. London: HMSO.

Department of Health (1991). *Dietary reference values for food energy and nutrients for the United Kingdom*. Report of the Panel on Dietary Reference Values of the Committee on Medical Aspects of Food Policy. Report on Health and Social Subjects No. 41. London: HMSO.

Department of Health (1992a). *The nutrition of elderly people*. Report of the Working Group of the Committee on Medical Aspects of Food Policy. Report on Health and Social Subjects No. 43. London: HMSO.

Department of Health (1992b). *The health of the nation: a strategy for health in England*. London: HMSO.

Department of Health (1994a). *Weaning and the weaning diet*. Report of the Working Group on the Weaning Diet of the Committee on Medical Aspects of Food Policy. Report on Health and Social Subjects No. 45. London: HMSO.

Department of Health (1994b). *Nutritional aspects of cardiovascular disease*. Report of the Cardiovascular Review Group Committee on Medical Aspects of Food Policy. Report on Health and Social Subjects No. 46. London: HMSO.

Department of Health (1997). *Nutritional aspects of the development of cancer*. Report of the Cancer Review Group of the Committee of Medical Aspects of Food and Nutrition Policy. Report on Health and Social Subjects No. 48. London: HMSO.

Health Education Authority (1995). *The balance of good health: information for educators and communicators*. London: Health Education Authority.

Acknowledgements

We should like to thank our colleagues, Dr Rory Williams, Dr Helen Bush and Mrs Anne Ellaway, MRC Medical Sociology Unit, Glasgow University, for their help with references. Mrs Janie Ferguson at Glasgow University Library helped with computer-based searches. Members of the Department of Human Nutrition, Glasgow University offered technical help and also provided us with references. Dr Marie Reid, then in the Department of Nutrition, Caledonian University, Glasgow, made helpful suggestions and confirmed decisions about exclusions.

We are grateful to the following: Professor Annie Anderson, School of Management and Consumer Studies, Dundee University, who offered advice and material and Dr Kathryn Backett-Milburn, Research Unit in Health and Behavioural Change, Edinburgh University, who provided references and support.

We should also like to acknowledge the contribution of Dr Lydia Martens, Department of Applied Social Science, Stirling University, who provided us with some material from some recent research and Professor Anne Murcott, Department of Social Sciences, South Bank University, London, who offered advice and practical help.

Ms Nikki Kidd contributed to the section entitled 'The social context of women's lives' and we are grateful to her.

This work received funding from the Department of Health; the views expressed in this publication are those of the authors and not necessarily those of the Department of Health.

1. Executive summary

Objectives

To review the opportunities for, and barriers to, dietary change among four groups identified in the Department of Health's document *R and D priorities in nutrition*; these four groups were 'healthy' women of childbearing age, women, infants aged under 1 year and children aged between 1 and 5 years.

To identify from the research literature any cultural, behavioural or societal opportunities for, and barriers to, good nutritional health which might inform policy by pointing to new ways of formulating or delivering interventions aimed at improving eating behaviour and nutritional status in these target groups.

To identify weaknesses and gaps in the existing literature.

To identify data for possible secondary analysis and to comment on the quality of literature in these fields.

Methods

A search of the literature was carried out between June and December 1996 covering the four subject areas using detailed specific criteria for inclusion of studies and for electronic databases, sets of key and mesh words to identify the studies.

The search included the disciplines of medicine and nursing, sociology, psychology, anthropology and nutrition, and the literature from health promotion. Sources other than journal articles were searched using other techniques.

The large number of studies initially identified were subsequently reduced, using a two-stage exclusion process.

Results

The searches yielded studies in each of the four groups.

Each contained studies using a range of research methods although fewer studies using qualitative methods were identified overall.

Studies were divided into two main categories: those reporting upon access factors and those reporting upon knowledge, culture and attitudes.

Women of childbearing age

The literature focuses upon access problems rather than opportunities; middle-class women have greater opportunities of access to superstores with a wide range of foods, due to ease of transport; because cost is of less importance and food storage is not a problem, food can be purchased in bulk.

The more extensive literature concentrates upon the barriers to good nutritional practices of women living in material deprivation where access, cost and storage are all problems. Studies of food availability and cost across neighbourhoods in the UK have emphasised that considerable variation does exist with better provision giving preference to middle-class neighbourhoods.

Women who live in material deprivation are shown to adopt 'safe' food purchasing strategies which may be seen as barriers to good nutrition as they inhibit purchasing of a greater range of foods.

Purchasing of certain foods is not only constrained by cost; research shows that attitudes to certain foods (for example some vegetables) contribute to a narrow diet and ways of creating greater familiarity with other reasonable cost foods may form a useful intervention.

One barrier to home cooking is the variety of dry ingredients required to cook and the need for cooking equipment as well as cooking skills. Home cooking interventions need to be tailored to show women how to prepare recipes to suit the available equipment and to reduce recipes to few ingredients.

Interventions might be directed not only to women but also to the males of the household; future trends in the division of labour (for example through more women working) may lead to males in the household being more likely to be allocated a major role in food preparation and home cooking.

Given the projections for greater participation by women in the labour market the workplace should be seen as an increasingly significant source of women's nutritional intake in the future and an important venue for nutritional interventions.

At present there is insufficient literature on the topic of eating out and eating fast foods, although in themselves these practices constitute neither an opportunity nor a barrier. There is evidence that the types of food which are currently 'eaten out' especially by young women (and men) tend to be less nutritious; nevertheless there are opportunities to change dietary behaviour in relation to the popular activity of 'eating out'.

Food choices privilege male partners and children and meal composition is decided by all family members (including small children); interventions regarding good nutritional practices should therefore be aimed at male partners and children in the family.

Although there is little research on the topic it is evident that snacking is a form of food consumption popular with particular groups (for example adolescents). The potential for dietary change should be recognised; at present snacking involves less nutritious groups of foods but the range of 'snacks' could be broadened.

The importance of a 'proper meal' is an opportunity to provide families with a variety of vegetables along with other food groups.

An interest in vegetarianism is apparent especially in young women and men and is linked to an interest in 'health'.

When investigating dietary change it is important not to isolate and focus upon specific nutritional changes but to understand that beliefs and attitudes towards certain foods may belong to broader 'cultural packages'.

Pregnant women

The majority of studies of pregnant women derived from the disciplines included in the search have not looked at the nutritional aspects of pregnancy.

Women see pregnancy as an opportunity for dietary change. Interventions could build upon this by targeting women in early pregnancy to encourage dietary change.

Many women are receptive to professional advice in pregnancy and the increased contact which women have with health professionals during pregnancy creates a period of opportunity for professionals.

Many professionals have some general knowledge about nutritional issues in pregnancy but lack specific knowledge, especially in relation to folate. More training in nutrition among professional groups (midwives, nursing staff, dietitians) which have high contact with women would be a useful intervention.

Women's knowledge of specific nutritional issues, especially the role of folate early in pregnancy, is evident.

Infants under 1

There is a large literature on breastfeeding which is predominantly quantitative and in which women's personal experiences and problems are seldom articulated 'in their own voice'.

Breastfeeding rates did not change over the ten-year period between 1980 and 1990 and the literature does not provide much evidence about how to facilitate an improvement in rates.

Hospital practices are important influences and many hospitals have introduced a number of changes to encourage breastfeeding. The literature highlights the variation in hospital practices that still exists and the variation in staff attitudes towards the value of breastfeeding. More attention should be directed towards nursing and midwifery staff to understand why these views are still held.

The literature emphasises the finding that breastfeeding is practised more by middle-class, older, better educated mothers who hold more positive attitudes to the practice. Barriers to successful breastfeeding are more likely to be cultural than practical although many women report practical problems in establishing and maintaining breastfeeding.

Interventions could be designed to change the negative views about breastfeeding in public places held by the 'general public'.

Many women wean their children earlier than official recommendations; little research exists on the topic of social and cultural attitudes towards weaning.

Mothers are thoughtful about the diet of their infants; this should form a positive basis for further education. Mothers do not necessarily understand the underlying nutritional messages regarding an infant's diet and the literature documents many examples of infants being fed inappropriate foods for their age.

Professional help is not always seen as appropriate. Different forms of professional interventions could be tried in order to increase legitimacy of the advice for some mothers.

Children aged 1–5 years

Much of the literature on children's food preferences and dislikes derives from psychological studies; the cultural context of children's eating patterns and meals is seldom examined although its importance is recognised.

There is evidence that children's food choices can be influenced by changing the food messages shown on television and the *potential* for change should make children's television an important forum for future interventions.

Food preferences are developed at an early age. Young children are an important target group for health interventions which help create positive eating habits at this early age.

Young children do not always understand food messages in the way that they are intended (for example the meaning of the term fat).

Lay nutritional knowledge is not always congruent with official recommendations and more understanding of mothers' beliefs is important.

With young children opportunities lie in the identification of positive rewards with eating, but conversely problems may arise when food is used as a form of control.

Mothers who supervise the food intake more closely may be providing an opportunity for the child to develop good nutritional behaviour.

1. Background

1. Introduction

This report is concerned with opportunities for, and barriers to, healthy eating in four target groups within the population: women of childbearing age; those who are pregnant; infants under the age of 1 year; and young children aged between 1 and 5 years. The report reviews research studies in order to identify opportunities for, and barriers to, dietary change.

The review covers research from a number of disciplines which have contributed to our understanding of nutritional health. This is strengthened by the range of research methods which have been used to tackle topics concerned with current dietary practices, attitudes and beliefs and to identify sources of potential dietary changes. Despite the apparent wealth of research, there remain striking omissions which are summarised within the text.

2. The target groups in context

(i) Women of childbearing age

The first group identified by the Department of Health's document *R and D priorities in nutrition* is women of childbearing age, defined for the review as women between the ages of 16 and approximately 50 (i.e. the menopause). Women between these ages are of considerable significance when considering dietary change, as they play a central role in caring, not only for themselves but also for their family (Graham, 1984). Sociological work, in particular, has provided accounts of the lives of families with children and a range of studies have noted the key role of women in looking after the family's nutritional needs (Murcott, 1983; Mayall, 1986; Charles and Kerr, 1988). The division of labour is such that women remain the family members most likely to prepare and cook the family meals. Targeting women provides the key to the nutritional health of all family members, and dietary change needs to be informed by an understanding of both the opportunities which are available to and the barriers which face women as central members of the household.

In spite of their greater life expectancy, there is good evidence, both self-reported and from community surveys, that women experience more ill health than men (Doyal, 1995). It is, however, increasingly accepted that good nutrition plays an important part in the prevention of many of the leading causes of illness and death in women (for example coronary heart disease, stroke, breast and bowel cancer, osteoporosis and diabetes) (Department of Health, 1991; Scottish Office, 1993). The diet-related Health of the Nation targets for the whole population, and recommendations for the healthy eating, which are summarised in the Foreword, are applicable to this group.

As well as the smaller-scale studies reviewed below, a number of large-scale government surveys provide a basis for our understanding of women's food intake (Gregory *et al.*, 1990; the National Food Surveys (NFS) 1994; 1995), although not all provide gender differentiated statistics (for example the NFS). The National Food Survey data are quoted in this review, however, as providing data on general trends in eating habits from a large number of British households. Gender-based statistics are available from the *Dietary and Nutritional Survey of British Adults* (Gregory *et al.*, 1990), a national survey of adults living in private households in Britain. Data from this survey indicate that women were more likely than men to consume high fibre, low fat foods (for example, more fresh fruit, cottage cheese, yoghurt and to drink skimmed milk), a finding replicated in smaller-scale studies (for example Anderson, Macintyre and West, 1994). Nevertheless the same national survey provided information showing that fat intake for the majority of women was over the target set by the Department of Health, being 39.2% of total energy intake (Gregory *et al.*, 1990), and singling out the younger age group (16–24) as least likely to eat many of the reduced fat or high fibre foods. In a supplement on 'Eating out', the survey also showed that it is women in the youngest age group who gain the greatest proportion of their total energy intake from eating out (Gregory *et al.*, 1990).

It is important to note the different ways of reporting of food intakes in the studies reviewed below; many studies take a 'food' or 'food groups'-based approach rather than a nutritional approach to eating habits. In some cases, family meals are discussed using only the broadest descriptive terms ('meat and vegetables', 'fruit and vegetables') rather than defining the nutritional intake of fibre, carbohydrates and proteins.

Social class variations have been illustrated in mortality as well as morbidity statistics (for example dental caries) (Department of Health, 1992; Scottish Office, 1993) and are important when discussing barriers to good nutritional health. Gregory *et al.* (1990) do indicate some class variations in eating habits, for example, that foods eaten by women in social classes I and II had a higher protein content than foods eaten by women in the other social classes (Gregory *et al.*, 1990)

(ii) Pregnant women

Pregnant women are important to this review for several reasons. As a category, they were excluded from the MAFF dietary and nutritional survey of adults since their dietary and nutritional status differed from those of other adults and they formed too small a group for separate analysis (Gregory *et al.,* 1990). Relatively little is known about the eating habits of pregnant women, although a number of small-scale studies (Anderson, Campbell and Shepherd, 1993; Schofield, Wheeler and Stewart, 1987) suggest that pregnant women see this time as one of opportunity for dietary change. The diet-related Health of the Nation targets and recommendations for healthy eating which are summarised in the Foreword apply to this group. In addition, women who are planning a pregnancy are recommended to consume additional folate, prior to conception and during the first 12 weeks of pregnancy by eating more folate-rich foods and taking a daily dietary supplement of 0.4 mg folic acid (Expert Advisory Group, 1992). The literature (although little current work) suggests uneven knowledge and adoption of the recommendations by health professionals and consumers. A number of the studies reviewed here were carried out prior to the publication of these Department of Health recommendations on folate intake in pregnancy.

The health of women is now also understood to play a part in the health status of the next generation. Although controversial (for example see Lucas, 1994), Barker (1994) and others (Wynn *et al.*, 1994) have stressed that the pre-pregnant status of a woman may show a generational effect in predisposing her children to heart disease and other risk factors such as high blood pressure (Barker, 1994). However, an interest in 'pre-pregnancy' (or 'preconception') has yet to become a well established research topic outside the medical literature.

(iii) Infants under 1

The Department of Health recommends that breastfeeding is maintained for 4 months, that no solid food is given before 4 months, and that a mixed diet should be introduced by 6 months (Department of Health, 1994). There is now a wealth of literature on infant feeding, much of which suggests that infant feeding practices are highly variable within the UK and that much conflicts with government recommendations, notably those on breastfeeding (Department of Health and Social Security, 1988; Department of Health, 1994).

Data from two national surveys provide a sound basis for understanding mothers' infant feeding practices, in both liquid and solid feeding. One series of studies on infant feeding in Great Britain from the Office of Population Censuses and Surveys (OPCS)* has been carried out for

*Now the Office for National Statistics (ONS)

more than fifteen years, the first survey taking place in 1975 (Martin, 1978), thus providing the basis for comparative analysis. The most recent survey (White, Freeth and O'Brien, 1992) demonstrated that over a ten-year period (1980–1990) there was virtually no change in the rate of breastfeeding, with 63% women reporting starting breastfeeding in 1990 compared with 65% mothers starting breastfeeding in 1980. Class and regional variations in breastfeeding (and infant solid feeding) were noted in the study and are reviewed further in the literature below.

Weaning has been defined as the expansion of an infant's diet to include foods and drinks other than breast and formula milks (Department of Health, 1994). Both the OPCS studies and a further survey funded by MAFF (Mills and Tyler, 1992) report on infant feeding and weaning by mothers. The study funded by MAFF surveyed the diets of nearly 500 infants aged between 6 and 12 months with mothers keeping a detailed seven-day diary and being personally interviewed. The OPCS study (Department of Health, 1994) and the MAFF-funded study (Mills and Tyler, 1992) report a range of weaning and infant feeding practices some of which do not conform to government recommendations. Apart from early weaning and infants being given family foods (chips, meats) a minority of infants were fed foods which were inappropriate to their age, for example, some infants were fed cows' milk.

(iv) Children 1–5

This is an age group which has reached the attention of the media and retail food markets in recent years and research reviewed below suggests that young children may have a strong influence upon their own food choices. Despite the increasing recognition of the potential role that young children may play in making their own food choices, the nutritional patterns of children in this age group have been neglected until recently when the National Diet and Nutrition Survey: children aged 1½–4½ (NDNS) was published (Gregory *et al.*, 1995). This survey was commissioned jointly by the Department of Health and MAFF to provide information about pre-school children living in private households in Britain. Few gender differences were reported in the survey (although boys were found to eat more fibre-related foods than girls). However, very clear social class variations emerged, with children from non-manual backgrounds being more likely to eat diets which were higher in fibre, protein and lower in fats (Gregory *et al.*, 1995).

Overall the study showed that the large majority of children ate a diet satisfactory in protein although over half did not eat eggs (54%), coated or fried fish (62%) or fish in any other way (62%). Their diet was higher in sugars than the recommended 10% of total dietary intake for this age group, with a mean average for children aged 2½–3½ of 19.3% and notably higher for boys than girls especially in the oldest age group (3½–4½) (Gregory *et al.*, 1995). Iron intake for the younger age groups was low, 77% of the RNI for those age groups but for the oldest age group, 4 years and upwards, the percentage was 96% of the RNI (Gregory *et al.*, 1995).

The NDNS survey forms a sound basis for understanding eating patterns of pre-school children. By contrast, much of the research reported below does not examine dietary intake of young children but considers in more detail the ways in which children's food preferences are shaped.

One requirement of this review was that it should establish, where possible, social variations in nutritional patterns as well as attitudes to and beliefs about foods. This has proved more difficult than anticipated; with the exception of the literature on breastfeeding which shows very clear social class differences, many of the studies reported below focus either upon gender or upon class (although occasionally both), while some include neither in their analyses (notably the literature on the final section, children aged 1–5 years). Some studies are US-based and do not consider class although they may use an associated measure of education, while for some topics, strong class differences are not apparent.

3. Search strategy

The objective of the search strategy was to carry out a systematic review of the relevant literature on women of childbearing age, pregnant women, infants under the age of 1 and children aged between 1 and 5 years. An outline of the strategy is described below, with details presented in Appendix C.

Initially the search presented certain challenges to the reviewers because of the breadth of the topics and the range of apparently relevant work in each field. The literature relevant to the four subjects reviewed below was known to span at least four major disciplines (medicine, psychology, sociology and anthropology) and within each, a variety of approaches was identified reflecting the methodologies acceptable within each discipline.

Sources for the review

- Electronic computerised databases – Medline (Index Medicus National Library of Medicine USA), EMBASE (Excerpta Medica) through BIDS, PsychLIT (American Psychological Association) for the medical and psychological references; IBSS, ASSIA (Abstracts in Social Sciences), for the sociological and anthropological sources. ACOMPLINE was also searched.

- Randomised controlled trials were identified through Medline and the Cochrane Data Base of Systematic Reviews.

- Other midwifery/consumer literature was identified through MIDIRS (Midwifery Information and Resource Service).

- Higher degree dissertations were identified through Dissertation Abstracts and through requesting known relevant theses.

- The Health Education Board for Scotland database was an important source, although the references showed a bias towards intervention studies.

- CRIB (Current Research In Britain).

- Books/book chapters; the social sciences, in particular, still publishes research findings in the form of book chapters, collected editions and ethnographies. There are fewer systematic ways in which to search book titles.

Books were identified in three ways:

- by feeding in key words into the computerised university library system which has a 'topic' index
- by following up references from important articles
- by word of mouth.

A number of experts in the field were consulted (see Appendix D for list); these experts provided further references, clarified issues and pointed us to other work in the field.

Although it had been intended to include studies from the 'grey' literature, the majority were concerned with health promotion activities and interventions and ultimately not included in the search as they were deemed to be beyond the scope of the review.

Inclusion criteria

- All studies included in this review were published between *January 1980 and December 1996 inclusive.*

- The search included only literature published *in the English language* (or with a full English abstract).

- Studies reporting upon research carried out in the *UK, North America, Australia, and other European countries.* Since the review has a strong bias in some sections towards 'knowledge, culture and attitudes' it was felt appropriate only to include studies which related to countries which might be seen to have some cultural similarities; priority was given to UK studies.

- Studies which fulfilled the *minimum methodological criteria* for inclusion (see Appendix C).

- Studies which included any of the sub-groups defined *by age or pregnancy* (see Appendix C).

Detailed criteria (see Appendix C) were defined in order to identify the relevant studies and to exclude those not appropriate to the review. Each of the included studies has been through this process and is reviewed both in the text below, and in the tables which appear in Appendix E using a pro forma agreed by the project team. For this purpose, each study has been referenced using the computer software Reference Manager, and in the tables the study methods are described in more detail than was possible in the text.

4. The social context of women's lives

As stated above, the central role of women in relation to eating habits and eating patterns in the family is evident in many studies which are examined in this report. However, women's role in the UK is not static and national surveys document the major trends in women's lives. Several issues have been selected as they have a direct impact on opportunities for, and barriers to, good nutritional health of two groups considered in this review, namely women of childbearing age and pregnant women.

Women are now living longer. Life expectancy for women remains higher than that for men, at 79 years (73 for men). They are also giving birth at a later age (Central Statistical Office, 1995). The mean age of childbearing has increased from 26.2 years in 1971 to 28.1 in 1993 and projections suggest that the mean will remain at this higher age (Central Statistical Office, 1994). The majority of women still give birth, although the average number of children per mother has dropped over the last two decades in all European countries. The UK figure of 1.8 children per mother is now the second highest in the EU (Central Statistical Office, 1995).

Three demographic trends are significant to this review. Single parent households are on the increase, with 14.8% of households with dependent children being headed by the natural mother only and 1.4% with the natural father only (the latter group increasing more rapidly) (Central Statistical Office, 1995). The proportion of families headed by a lone parent has increased steadily over the last quarter century with, in

1992, one in five mothers with dependent children being a lone mother (Central Statistical Office, 1995).

Many of these single parents with dependent children live in considerable hardship (Graham, 1993), with 90% of single mothers receiving Income Support as do 50% divorced/separated mothers (Central Statistical Office, 1994; Dowler and Calvert, 1995). Until recently little systematic research has been carried out on nutritional deprivation among low-income groups in the UK (Dowler and Calvert, 1995). Both Dowler and Calvert and others have studied the eating patterns and food choice of women (and their dependants) living on a low income, concluding that many of those living in deprivation have a diet which is often monotonous and narrow (for example HEA, 1989; Dobson *et al.*, 1994; Dowler and Calvert, 1995). A number of studies are reviewed below which focus upon this group of women and their children.

Two further demographic trends are related and relevant. There has been an increase in the number of women who remain childless, with projections suggesting that this group of women will increase (Central Statistical Office, 1995). The interpretation of this finding is not straightforward when considering their nutritional status and domestic responsibilities. Childless women may live with and be responsible for others, or may live singly. Research has not explored these different scenarios and the implications for women's general and nutritional wellbeing of these different lifestyles.

Related to this, there has been an increase in the number of single person households as a proportion of all households; although the increase is greatest for men under pensionable age there is also a growing number of women in this category (Central Statistical Office, 1995). This is a group of women neglected by those interested in women and nutritional health; none of the studies reviewed relates to this group of women and little is known about their socioeconomic status, their eating patterns or the opportunities their domestic situation provides for nutritional health.

The final trend is also central to this review although to date it remains an area grossly neglected by researchers of all disciplines. Although much of the literature assumes that women will continue to play a central nurturing role within the household (Graham, 1993), statistics suggest otherwise. Recent figures chart the rise in economic activity of women in the paid labour market; of all women aged 16 and over, 43.9% were economically active in 1971, 52.6% in 1993 and 56% (projected) in 2006 (Central Statistical Office, 1995). Women are becoming employed in both full-time and part-time work, with more working full-time (6 165 000 women full-time compared with 5 045 000 working part time) (Central Statistical Office, 1994).

Important, too, are the data which report that an increasing number of women are entering higher education and joining the professions. Thus the proportion of all higher education students (full- and part-time) who are female has risen within a relatively short period, with 40% female in 1984/85 rising to 47% in 1992/93 (Department for Education and Employment, 1996). The number of female postgraduates has risen strikingly over the last decade from 6% in 1985/86 to 21% in 1992/93 (AUT statistics).

Despite the rising numbers of women in paid work, major changes in the sharing of household duties have not been recorded over the last fifteen years. One significant example is that of household shopping with only a slightly greater proportion of households reporting this to be a shared task in 1991 than in 1983 (47% v. 44%) (Central Statistical Office, 1995), although research reviewed in this report comments further on this finding. Making the evening meal remains very much a woman's task with fewer doing it in more recent times (70% in 1991 compared to 77% in 1983). Other tasks seen as carried out by 'mainly women' are washing and ironing, household cleaning and looking after sick children (Central Statistical Office, 1995).

2. Results

1. Introduction

Presentation of the results of this review has been divided into three main subgroups; the literature relating to women of childbearing age and pregnant women is reviewed first, followed by a second section which deals with infants under the age of 1 year. Finally, the review focuses upon the literature concerned with young children aged between 1 and 5 years. Within each subgroup, there are two basic sections. The first sections review literature relating to 'access' issues which includes geographical access as well as access issues which may involve barriers to dietary change because of material deprivation. The second sections are entitled 'knowledge, culture and attitudes', and focus upon studies which have identified broadly 'cultural' issues which provide opportunities for, or barriers to, dietary change. For the purposes of the review the literature has been grouped in this way, but it is noted in the text that some studies of women and young children cross these subgroups and are reviewed in two subsections, while some studies report upon both 'access' and 'cultural' issues and likewise are reviewed in both sections.

2. Women of childbearing age and pregnant women

Access

(i) Women of childbearing age

The 'access' literature is broad and methodologically diverse. Studies range from those initiated by the food industry to report on trends in eating patterns (London Food Commission, undated) to those concerned with a detailed description of barriers to nutrition in subgroups of the population, such as mothers living on a low income (see, for example, Dobson *et al.*, 1994).

When studying the barriers and opportunities related to access issues, it must be noted that the literature focuses overwhelmingly upon the difficulties of access, with a number of studies funded specifically to identify nutritionally related concerns about low-income mothers and their children (for example LIPT, 1996; Dobson *et al.*, 1994; Dowler and Calvert, 1995). Indeed, the lack of literature which takes a representative sample of the population is notable and far less is reported about middle-class eating patterns.

This section is methodologically varied. The 'shopping basket' approach, analysing food availability and purchasing, is commonly used in identifying foods bought (Welsh Consumer Council, 1993) although seldom relating this to food consumption. A few studies have used mixed methods, combining an analysis of foods consumed with further information derived from consumer questionnaires, while a few studies (for example Dowler and Calvert, 1995) combine these data with those derived from interviews of a sample of the respondents. Only a small number (Dowler and Calvert, 1995; Charles and Kerr, 1988) report on domestic decision-making within the home and the kind of in-depth decision-making which results in the purchase of certain foods. Likewise although the majority of visits to the supermarket involve the use of cars, there is little evidence about who drives the car or who accompanies the driver. The influence of these factors is virtually ignored (but see Charles and Kerr, 1988).

Distribution and availability of food shops

The London Food Commission (LFC) described three major changes that have taken place in the structure of the food retail industry since the early 1950s (LFC, undated). First, there has been a growing dominance of a small number of large multiple groups. Secondly, the size of individual stores or superstores has increased considerably. Finally, there has been a substantial decline in the total number of food retail outlets. The Low Income Project Team report (LIPT, 1996) supports these trends identified in the 1980s with recent data showing that the number of food retail outlets decreased by 35% between 1980 and 1992 from 121 600 to 78 606, mainly at the expense of small grocery outlets and specialist shops such as butchers and greengrocers. On the other hand, the average store size increased from 6924 sq. ft in 1980 to 12 850 sq. ft in 1994 (LIPT, 1996).

The Low Income Project Team identify further trends, notably that the proportion of shopping journeys by car has increased from 44.9% in 1975/76 to 64.1% in 1991/93, and the average distance has increased from 13.7 miles in 1989/91 to 15.3 miles in 1991/93. Only 20% of shopping journeys are on foot, while 12% are by bus (LIPT, 1996). Government data provide information on car ownership, reporting that in 1991 45% of households had one car and 32% of households were without regular use of a car (Central Statistical Office, 1994). It is not clear, however, how many women have access to a car for shopping. Data reported in *Social Trends* indicate that many women do not possess a full driving licence; combined data between 1991 and 1993 show that just over half (53%) the female population aged 17 and over possessed a full driving licence while the figure for men was 81% (Central Statistical Office, 1995).

Division of labour within the household relating to food shopping

Although a weekly task for most households, little research has been carried out upon the division of labour in relation to food shopping. In one of the few studies on women and food beliefs and practices which took a qualitative approach (and therefore where the respondents were able to raise issues important to them), Charles and Kerr's respondents talked about shopping (Charles and Kerr, 1988). The authors report from their sample of 200 women that it was usually the woman in the household who made the decision about what foods to buy. About half reported help with the shopping, thus 41% did most of the shopping with some help from their partner (for example the partner driving them to the supermarket) and 10.5% shared the task with their male partner; just under half of the sample (46%) said that they were wholly responsible for the shopping (Charles and Kerr, 1988).These proportions were very similar to the findings from Calnan's qualitative study with a small sample who were asked about the same issue (Calnan, 1990).

Warde and Hetherington's survey was conducted with a different sample, which was older, more affluent and living in larger households (Warde and Hetherington, 1994). The researchers asked a slightly different question, namely 'who did the task last', noting that the more general question about who *usually* does the task 'underestimates women's actual contribution'. In the questionnaire responses from couple households, a larger proportion (30%) of their sample reported that they shared the shopping. Fifty-four per cent reported that women did the shopping and 14% reported that men did the main shopping (Warde and Hetherington, 1994).

These findings are important in that they suggest that it is increasingly difficult to shop in large superstores with their broader range of foods, without making a long journey. Private transport facilitates the travel, but access to a car (or a driver) is not available to all women. As Charles and Kerr note, 'Class profoundly influences . . . the options that are open to (women) in terms of providing food for their family' (Charles and Kerr, 1988, p.167). The existing research indicates a situation of inequality; superstores represent opportunities to those with direct or indirect access to private transport, and a barrier to those for whom transport – public or private – is not easily available.

Inequalities in the availability of certain foods

There are a number of studies which have reviewed the relationship between retail access, cost and range of foods available in different areas within cities. These studies have been carried out across the UK (England, Wales and Scotland) and in general have concluded that the availability and cost of foods does vary within cities, with a bias towards greater availability of varied, fresh and proportionately cheaper foods, in higher income areas. The methodological problems in carrying out these studies have been noted by every author.

Several large-scale surveys have noted regional variations in food consumption, as well as recording gender difference (for example the National Food Survey). Whichelow and her colleagues, reporting findings from the Health and Lifestyle Survey (carried out in 1984/85), note for example, that there are significant differences across the 11 regions in relation to the consumption of chips and fried foods, fruit and salad (Whichelow, Erzinelioglu and Cox, 1991). Analyses of gender differences reveal that women were more likely than men to eat fruit, salads and fruit juice 'frequently' and to choose 'brown' bread and skimmed milk, and less likely to eat potatoes, pulses, processed meats, eggs, chips and fried foods (Whichelow, Erzinelioglu and Cox, 1991). Issues about gender and attitudes towards food are discussed in this chapter (pp. 35–49). Other studies, however, have explored the variation in availability of food across regions in some detail.

In a pilot study, the London Food Commission (LFC) investigated the differences between food retail outlet prices in London (LFC, undated). They reported that the price difference of 31 items between the cheapest superstore and the most expensive small supermarket was just under 21%. Victor Value (the Tesco-owned discount store) proved cheaper than both Tesco stores and superstores by around 10% but carried only half the range of survey items available at the Tesco superstore and almost 40% fewer items than at the Tesco store of comparable size. The LFC study noted the bulk of foods available at Victor Value was processed and that it stocked no fresh vegetables and had a very poor range of fish and cheese products. This study notes that the retail strategy of investing in superstores for affluent, car-borne shoppers has resulted in a polarisation of types of food product available and a trend towards unequal access to nutritious food products with shoppers with restricted income and mobility being limited to high street discount stores (LFC, undated).

The Welsh Consumer Council carried out a survey to establish prices and availability of foodstuffs in different types of shops and areas in Wales (Welsh Consumer Council, 1993). They surveyed cost and availability of 30 items from a sample of 111 shops (quality was not assessed), and reported that the survey findings confirmed that smaller shops generally charged higher prices than large shops and that the cost of the selected items was 11.2% more expensive than in large shops. Geographical variations in price differences between North and South Wales were more marked in large shops, with prices tending to be lower in the South. The survey also highlighted the difficulties with such apparently straightforward comparisons, as some small shops were affiliated to larger chains (which affected pricing), not all items were available for comparison in each shop and pricing variations sometimes depended upon the shop's definition of certain foods (for example 'lean' beef) (Welsh Consumer Council, 1993).

A methodologically similar exercise ('the shopping basket approach') was carried out in Glasgow on a smaller scale, as part of the West of Scotland Twenty-07 study, by Sooman, Macintyre and Anderson (1993). The researchers also note the limitations of such a method, which does not report on what individuals eat, merely what is available in food shops. The difficulty, too, of comparing items in terms of weight, quality, quantity, size and brand presents further challenges. Sooman and her colleagues found that not only were 'healthy foods' (their term) more available in the middle-class area of Glasgow but their cost was greater in a more socially disadvantaged area than in a more affluent area (Sooman, Macintyre and Anderson, 1993). Mooney, using the same approach, also came to similar conclusions in a smaller London-based study (Mooney, 1990).

Sooman's team focused upon the lack of availability of what the authors term 'healthy foods' in socioeconomically deprived areas (Sooman, Macintyre and Anderson, 1993). They also noted the good availability of fresh fish and fruit and vegetables in middle-class areas, the prices for the items being slightly cheaper in the more middle-class area of the city. In a related project, Forsyth and colleagues included questions about foods consumed in different neighbourhoods by individuals belonging to two age cohorts (40 years and 60 years old) of the West of Scotland Twenty-07 longitudinal study (Forsyth, Macintyre and Anderson, 1994). The authors report variation between neighbourhoods on certain items, with more fruit and vegetables, brown or wholemeal bread, high fibre cereals and spreading fats (polyunsaturated fatty acids) consumed in 'middle-class' neighbourhoods. The researchers also found variations by gender (notably with salt intake being higher among males than females) and by age (Forsyth, Macintyre and Anderson, 1994).

Thus the *assumed* opportunity of good access to certain foods in higher income areas suggested by 'shopping basket' surveys is shown, in this study at least, to be a real opportunity for families in those areas. These studies on food availability also underline very heavily what appears to be a deliberate strategy of the retail market in terms of placing and pricing of foods in selected neighbourhoods. A large number of health promotion interventions have tried to redress the balance by making (for example) certain foods (grains, fruit and vegetables) more available in low-income areas through food co-operatives.

Food costs and family practices

As noted above, there is a tendency for research to focus upon the inequalities of access to food retail outlets by those on low incomes. A

UK series of methodologically strong studies have used a variety of research methods to provide greater evidence of the problems of 'access' to a varied diet (HEA, 1989; NCH, 1991; Dobson *et al.*, 1994; Dowler and Calvert, 1995). Dowler and Calvert (1995) combined qualitative and quantitative methods in their study of a cross-section of 200 lone parent households and also assessed the nutritional status of their sample through a dietary intake survey. This combination of methods allowed the researchers to conclude that those respondents (and their children) who exclusively used discount food shops (22% of the sample) had worse nutritional outcomes than those who used other shops as well or instead. The authors reported that they had no evidence that the quality of the food stuffs was bad in discount stores but that the range of foodstuffs may be more limited (Dowler and Calvert, 1995).

The Health Education Authority (HEA) study used both food diaries and interviews to understand food shopping behaviour in their sample of 47 low-income households (HEA, 1989). The qualitative approach makes the findings difficult to summarise briefly but included evidence that most respondents whose accommodation provided storage facilities shopped weekly or fortnightly at the cheapest store, reported frustrations at shopping on a low budget and focused upon purchasing familiar items (HEA, 1989).

However, the difficulty of travelling with young children without a car prevented many single parents in the sample from using the cheaper supermarkets or discount stores and led to an increased dependence upon local shops and nearby supermarkets, where they often had to pay higher prices. Small local shops were consistently reported to be the most expensive type of retail outlet and were only used by respondents for perishable items and in emergencies.

Dobson and her colleagues, among others, have found that price dominated decisions; families reported that foods such as meat, vegetables, fruit, staples and snacks were seen as essential items although salads and fresh fruit were regarded as luxury items (Dobson *et al.*, 1994). Likewise, respondents from the HEA study emphasised that income rather than taste was the barrier to purchasing certain foods (HEA, 1989). Dowler and Calvert (1995) on the other hand, have reported that family eating patterns resulted from a variety of factors, long-term poverty being one, but other commitments (for example, automatic deductions from benefits) also affecting food choice. These studies have all used interviews, and the lack of congruence between the findings is more likely to be because the researchers have raised different issues with their respondents. All studies confirm that price is an important factor in food purchasing.

Little US research has been identified which explores the issues tackled under 'access'; however, the work by Furst *et al.* (1996) is relevant here. The researchers carried out semi-structured interviews with 20 shoppers selected at random, the majority of whom were women (although the authors do not focus upon gender differences). The resultant model presented by the authors included five major categories of influences on food choice, resources and food context, which are relevant here.

In relation to 'resources', interviewees simply noted budgetary and other constraints relating to food purchase which included respondents noting problems of equipment and food storage. The authors also reported that resources varied over the life course, changing in importance as state of health, income and independence altered (Furst *et al.*, 1996). 'Food context' refers to the environment in which food was purchased (for example, purchasing particular foods which were on 'special offer') as well as the specific food supply factors such as seasonality. The authors note that what was locally available influenced an individual's food purchasing (Furst *et al.*, 1996). This study confirms UK findings, but through the model, provides a more theoretical approach to food choice.

Mooney (1990), in her 'shopping basket' study, estimated that a 'healthy diet' would cost around 42% of Income Support benefit per week for individuals aged 25 and over, whereas the cost of the 'less healthy diet' (items not meeting Food Health Policy Guidelines) was only around 25% of Income Support benefit (Mooney, 1990). Mooney comments on the difficulties of such a costing exercise, as already discussed.

Other studies, too, have underlined the cost of a 'healthy' diet (for example Cade and Booth, 1990). It is not surprising to find that those living on low incomes report diets which are deficient in a number of important nutrients. Dowler and Calvert (1995) found that those in the poorest households had a limited nutrient base, two or three foods providing the majority of a nutrient. Gibney and Lee (1993) found that women in their Irish sample from a locality with chronically high unemployment had low intakes of alcohol and fibre, and intakes of certain vitamins and minerals were lower than recommended levels. Cost and (lack of) availability were again given as the reasons for low fruit purchasing (Gibney and Lee, 1993). This study also emphasised the additional cost of feeding older children whose energy intakes were increasing.

In some of the above studies of women on low incomes, the researchers asked about the relationship between the pattern of family expenditure and food purchasing (NCH, 1991; Dobson *et al.*, 1994; Dowler and Calvert, 1995). These studies are rich in detail from the interviews and provide an in-depth understanding of the balancing of finances operated in these families. Regardless of the specific differences between the findings, each study suggests that food purchasing is but one of several 'priorities' for the families.

In the study by Dobson and her colleagues, for example, their respondents, all of whom were on very low incomes, reported that they aimed to spend money quickly after receipt of benefits on weekly or fortnightly food shopping to avoid it being 'frittered away' (Dobson *et al.*, 1994). The authors noted the flexible nature of food expenditure which varied depending upon the income of the week (Dobson *et al.*, 1994). Many of the lone parents in Dowler and Calvert's study also said that they gave precedence to paying bills over other expenditure, including food (Dowler and Calvert, 1995). As the authors conclude, the price of controlling expenditure was inadequacy of nutrient intake, poor food variety, and less nutritionally sound dietary patterns (Dowler and Calvert, 1995). Conversely, however, a small sample of parents drawn from 52 National Children's Homes centres, reported that they would not pay bills and risk getting into debt rather than go short of food (NCH, 1991).

A number of researchers (for example Murcott, 1983; Charles and Kerr, 1988; Dobson *et al.*, 1994) have argued that when resources are strained, eating patterns, as they have done for decades, privilege the men and children in the family with the women traditionally eating less and/or less 'high status food'. Dobson *et al.* (1994) and Dowler and Calvert (1995) both report strategies within families of some members going without food so that other family members could eat more. The survey section of the National Children's Homes study offers further support for the above findings. In this study 20% of parents reported that they had 'gone hungry' in the last month because of lack of money, and 44% had gone short of food in the last year to ensure that others in the family had enough to eat (NCH, 1991). One in 10 children under 5 had gone without food in the last month because of lack of money. Nearly 1 in 4 had gone without food during the last month because they did not like the food on offer (this aspect of family life will be discussed later in the report) (NCH, 1991).

In families of lower income, the possibility that the children might not like, and therefore would not eat, food is an inhibiting factor in purchasing novel foods (HEA, 1989; Dobson *et al.*, 1994). Dowler and Calvert report, in their study of low-income families, that those who regularly cooked from fresh or raw ingredients achieved greater dietary variety for themselves and their children but confirmed the findings of other studies (see 'Fruit and vegetable consumption', p.44) that those who did not experiment and who were more tied to their children's tastes, ended up with restricted diets (Dowler and Calvert, 1995). In the HEA study, the strategy was to buy more convenience foods which were seen as easier to budget for, relatively cheap, easy to prepare and popular with children. These factors however combined to produce a diet which tended to be repetitive and limited in variety (HEA, 1989). The pattern of food purchasing among single women was more varied and less planned than among families, and depended upon their age, type of accommodation, gender and social group. Nine of the single sample were living in bed and breakfast accommodation or bedsits and survey findings suggested that they tended to spend rather more on food than other respondents in the study, the main reason being their greater reliance upon relatively expensive take-aways, cafés and local shops.

The complex nature of decision-making about foods is further reported in Section 4. 'Children aged 1 to 5 years', but is already suggestive that *all* family members rather than parents alone, are influential in food purchasing. These findings about 'safe' food purchasing strategies, however, may be viewed as barriers in that they suggest that this factor inhibits purchasing of a greater range of foods.

The brief reference to 'single' women in the HEA study discussed above is interesting as this is a group to which almost no research attention has been directed, although the finding suggests that they have greater opportunities to change in dietary behaviours. Research with this group of women (not confined to those living in material deprivation) should be a priority area for the future, bearing in mind the difficulties in defining 'singleness' in our society.

Food preparation and the division of labour

Sociologists writing in this area have noted repeatedly that food production is intimately related to the social relations in society (Calnan, 1990), and the central location of women in the household (Graham, 1993) as providers of the family meal (Murcott, 1983). Murcott argues that while there is an *assumption* within society that women remain the managers of food provision in the household, there are indications that family eating patterns are more complex (Murcott, 1997). National studies such as the *Dietary and Nutritional Survey of British Adults* (Gregory *et al.*, 1990) report on the kinds of foods eaten in households, while the National Food Survey reports on foods consumed inside and outside the home. However, the manner in which these foods are constructed into meals, and by whom, remains little researched. In the systematic search for relevant studies for this review only a few studies were traced on home food preparation and family eating patterns.

Most studies in this broad field report that cooking (the definition of cooking is not usually specified but appears to include food preparation) is predominantly seen as a female activity (for example Backett, 1990; Murcott, 1983). The few studies which deal with men's involvement with cooking (for example Charles and Kerr, 1988; Backett, 1990; Warde and Hetherington, 1994) found that if men cooked it was seldom a routine event ('Most men in our sample only cooked as a standby or if they were particularly interested in food', Charles and Kerr, 1988, p. 45). Studies by Backett, and Warde and Hetherington confirm the finding that if men did cook it tended to be for special occasions such as dinner parties or barbecues, in which case the food prepared was special and very elaborate (Backett, 1990; Warde and Hetherington, 1994). Charles and Kerr, and Warde and Hetherington found social class differences with food preparation, with men in social classes I and II more likely to help with cooking than working-class men (Charles and Kerr, 1988; Warde and Hetherington, 1994). The extent to which domestic roles are still strongly gender specific is illustrated further by Hetherington and Warde who noted that if the meal involved buying a take-away or alcohol then the male partners were more likely to take responsibility (Warde and Hetherington, 1994).

However, some North American researchers (for example Olson, Ponzetti and Olsen, 1989; Blair and Lichter, 1991) have attempted to quantify time allocation of domestic tasks. Both these US studies indicate that food preparation is always a time-consuming task. Blair and Lichter's gender-based analysis shows clearly that women devote a greater proportion of the total time they spend on household tasks to those which are food-related than men do (women 28.7%; men 15.7%). By contrast, the proportions of time spent on food shopping were more equal (women 8.7%; men 9.1%) (Blair and Lichter, 1991).

Douthitt (1989) analysed data from a 1981 national sample of married Canadian men and women, to look at time use across a range of domestic tasks in the home, including food preparation. Her sample was further differentiated by employment status and the number of children (if any) in the household. The author found that employed married women with no children spent the highest proportion of all groups on food preparation in the home (31%), with the smallest proportion of time spent by women with children under 5 years (18%). A similar trend was found with women not in the labour force, with childless women spending 30% of time on food preparation compared to 20% of time by those with young children. Men with an employed wife and children under 5 spent the greatest proportion of time in food preparation (32%), followed by men with no children whose wives were in employment (13%). Men with young children and a wife not in the labour market spent the smallest proportion of their time in food preparation (9% of their time) (Douthitt, 1989).

These studies bring out the gender bias in food preparation, which is part of the more generalised caring tasks of women in the home, and attempt to quantify the time spent on various domestic tasks. However, the studies also begin to illustrate the factors which contribute to variation in time spent on the task (such as paid employment and dependent children). Contrary to what one might expect, it is those women who do not have children who spend more time on food preparation.

Home cooking

Home cooking, that is the preparation of meals from raw ingredients in the home, is a curiously neglected issue within the nutritional literature. The nutritional value of home cooked foods is seldom questioned and seldom researched, and few studies which deal with home cooking were located in any of the searches for this review. Although home cooked food is assumed to be nutritionally sound, only one study has been located which assesses the nutritional value of home cooked foods versus ready to eat meals, and this does not support the thesis of the superiority of home cooking (Anderson unpublished, cited in Scottish Office, 1993).

Home cooking is relevant here in as much as research highlights issues of cost and wastage (there is overlap with 'shopping behaviour' since shopping and cooking are obviously highly interdependent). Respondents in the HEA study (HEA, 1989) themselves raised the issue of cooking in the interviews, emphasising that price, speed of preparation and 'family acceptability' were the paramount concerns. Women who cooked more frequently were often more confident about tailoring complex recipes to suit their needs and reported sharing recipes with friends and family (HEA, 1989).

The majority of families in the HEA survey did have access to fridges and cookers but some of the single people did not (HEA, 1989). Freezers, often second-hand or shared, were used extensively by parents who had them and were an important factor in successful budgeting and planning. The NCH study reported on the lack of access to cookers (and cooking utensils) and to storage of food. Families without such facilities had a higher incidence of eating practices which involved less nutritious foods than those with access (NCH, 1991). These findings underline the material and practical barriers facing women and their families living in constrained circumstances, and the importance of having access to basic kitchen equipment for food preparation. Although there are few opportunities offered in such accommodation it is noted that where storage and refrigeration facilities were available these were heavily used.

In England and Wales changes imposed by the National Curriculum have resulted in 'optional subjects', such as the study of food, being excluded through lack of time and resources (Lang and Baker, 1993). From an unpublished study of skills of a sample of 7- to 15-year-olds (sample size not reported), it was found that 61% could program a video recorder, compared to 54% who could bake a cake. Thirty-eight per cent could cook a jacket potato in the oven (reported in Lang and Baker, 1993). However, about half the young people helped in the kitchen once a week or more and over fifty per cent knew how to slice, peel and grill

(National Food Alliance, and reported in Lang and Baker, 1993). The lack of cookery skills reported by young women has given rise to concern from health educationalists and has resulted in a number of intervention projects teaching cooking skills being set up in many regions in the UK.

Researchers from various disciplines (cultural studies, sociology and anthropology) have noted that foods have differing moral values in society (Murcott, 1983; Mayall, 1986; Fantasia, 1995). The unquestioned assumption that home cooking is morally superior is evident in Stitt and his colleagues' discussion paper on the loss of cooking skills. The authors argue, without presenting evidence in support of their claims, that the benefits of home cooking include offering greater choice, creativity, economy, control over diet, taste and freshness (Stitt, Jepson and Paulson-Box, 1995). This view is also held by respondents in Charles and Kerr's qualitative study leading the authors to comment 'Home cooking from fresh ingredients has a moral as well as nutritional value, it is part of being a good wife and mother' (Charles and Kerr, 1988, p. 129). By the same token, convenience foods were also seen as foods which were not fresh or natural (Charles and Kerr, 1988).

The pleasures of cooking are either under-reported or simply not studied. Little literature can be found which discusses this topic even tangentially. Only two studies (with different samples) reported conflicting responses from women about their views of home cooking. Female respondents from Warde and Hetherington's middle-class, slightly older sample rated cooking more highly than those from Charles and Kerr's study (Charles and Kerr, 1988; Warde and Hetherington, 1994).

The research on home cooking is intriguing although it lacks sufficient substance to be able to make clear statements about opportunities or barriers. There are not enough studies to allow comment on the nutritional value of home cooking but it is broadly accepted that home cooking is socially important and this should be seen as an opportunity for nutritional interventions. However, interventions relating to dietary change may wish to be concerned not only with women but also with the males of the household; future trends in the division of labour (for example through more women working) may lead to men (both sons and fathers) in the household being more likely to be allocated a major role in food preparation and home cooking.

Convenience foods

Social Trends data show that the purchasing of convenience foods rose by 10% in the decade to 1993 and is still rising (Central Statistical Office, 1995). Convenience foods themselves cannot be seen in terms of either an opportunity or a barrier. However, evidence that low-income mothers of young children appear to rely heavily on convenience foods such as burgers, fish fingers, sausages and pizzas rather than cooking from raw ingredients (HEA, 1989), implies that the less nutritious convenience foods form a significant proportion of the diet.

The reason that HEA study respondents gave for buying convenience foods was that the foods had become familiar to the family and that experimentation with unknown food could lead to wastage if the food was disliked. Convenience foods were reported to hold several advantages: they were quick and easy to prepare and less messy than cooking from raw (HEA, 1989). Little other research has reported specifically upon convenience foods as a nutritional option.

Eating out

While eating out, defined in the NFS as 'the consumption of food and drink eaten outside the home which is not obtained from the household's stocks' (MAFF, 1995, p. 39), is recognised by the food retail trade as a growing market, this is an area with little research evidence about the factors which affect consumer access to eating out. Although the NCH study notes that of the women in their low-income study, 40% said that eating take-away food was 'too costly' (NCH, 1991), few studies elaborate on who may eat out and under what circumstances (although see the work of Martens and Warde reviewed in 'Styles of eating – eating out and snacking' (p. 41). A brief discussion on possible barriers and opportunities is included, however, and eating out is identified as a significant area for further research.

The trend towards 'eating out' is noted in a number of publications (for example Gregory *et al.*, 1990; NFS, 1996), with both publications providing some information based on gender. 'Eating out' can be undertaken in a range of circumstances, including eating out at a restaurant as a social occasion and buying take-away foods, while workplace canteens are also important venues for an increasing number of meals consumed. The 1990 MAFF study reported that more men than women consume food outside the home, with 94% of men and 90% of women deriving some food energy out of the home during the 7-day study period. Men derived a greater proportion of their energy by eating out (Gregory *et al.*, 1990).

In an economic review of the catering market, Payne and Payne identify public houses as the largest sector in the eating out market (Payne and Payne, 1993). Burger bars, pizza houses and fish and chip shops account for over 25% of the eating out market with the first two categories enjoying considerable growth since the early 1980s (Payne and Payne, 1993). NFS figures indicate that in the categories 'eaten out' and 'take-away food', McDonald's is the market leader (in terms of annual revenue) although fish and chip shops and Chinese food also yield strong take-away sales (MAFF, 1995). Both Payne and Payne and the NFS have noted that the younger age group (aged 15–24 years) make most use of particular kinds of fast food establishments, notably those selling pizzas, fast food snacks and fish and chips (MAFF, 1995; Payne and Payne, 1993), with this age group also spending most on soft drinks and confectionery, biscuits, crisps and savoury snacks (MAFF, 1995).

Eating out and eating fast foods do not constitute an opportunity or a barrier in themselves and analysis of popular foods eaten out of the home indicates that there is considerable variation in the major food values of popular foods. Rees cites the energy value of burgers as varying by as much as 400%, with the fat content ranging between 35% and 66%, and having up to 1800 mg sodium (*Nutrition Action Newsletter* 1989, cited in Rees, 1992). However, a number of commentators have noted the high calorific value of many popular foods, which have high energy density, are high in fats (including saturated fats), sodium, sugar and additives and are low in fibre, vitamins and minerals (Rees, 1992; Lobstein, 1988; Heald and Felix, 1992).

Payne and Payne identify two significant trends in the food industry as 'convenience' and 'health' and comment specifically upon the health influence which, they write, 'Will be reflected in an increased offering of salads, low fat food, vegetarian meals and, perhaps, fresh and healthy ingredients' (Payne and Payne, 1993). Earlier US studies using data from cash registers of food purchased at restaurants (Wagner and Winett, 1988; Winett *et al.*, 1991) suggest that consumers are receptive to increases in the provision of healthier foods, although the marketing strategy has to be appropriate. More recent government documents also emphasise the trend towards the provision of good quality and a broad variety of food from retailers and restaurateurs (for example, Scottish Office, 1996). More research is required on the topic although the opportunity factor in changing dietary behaviour in relation to the popular activity of 'eating out' is considerable, and the Payne and Payne analysis suggests that the trends are positive.

Data from the NFS identify the workplace as the eating-out venue with the highest percentage of fat contribution to total energy of the food provided (NFS, 1996), with an average of 48% fat. Schools were placed second, with 42.8%, and restaurants, pubs and take-aways third with 40.3%. All values are higher than Department of Health recommendations. The figures are not broken down by gender and it is not known to what extent women are likely to partake of workplace meals. Given the projections for greater participation by women in the labour market one might highlight the workplace as an increasingly significant source of women's nutritional intake in the future and an important site for nutritional interventions.

Work and household eating patterns

At present, a limited number of research studies have been carried out specifically on the impact of working women on the household eating patterns; what little research exists is mainly from North America (for example Jensen, Rao and Hilton, 1989; Kim, 1989).

Taking a nutritional rather than a social perspective, Johnson and her colleagues studied the effect of mothers' employment on the quality of the diets of their young children (aged 2–5). Using parental recall of meals on four non-consecutive days, the researchers analysed the adequacy of the diets and concluded that mothers' employment (whether full- or part-time did not have a detrimental effect on their children's diets (Johnson, Smiciklas-Wright and Crouter, 1992). However, these apparently reassuring findings need to be placed in context. This US study focused upon a useful hypothesis but contained limitations in the sampling strategy which were acknowledged by the authors; furthermore, there was no attempt to compare these children's diets to those of non-working mothers with children of similar age, and the analysis in terms of employment level was rather basic.

Using US data collected in 1980 and (separately) 1986, Jensen and his colleagues reported few differences between working and non-working wives and few changes between the two surveys (Jensen, Rao and Hilton, 1989). They report that their finding that working wives disliked food shopping to a greater extent than non-working wives confirms earlier work. The researchers also noted that working women adopted time-saving strategies with regard to meal preparation (Jensen *et al.*, 1993).

Kim's analysis, using a nationwide Canadian survey data, looked at the effect of the wife's working status (non-working/working including part-time) on two sets of variables which included consumption frequency of 34 convenience foods and frequency of meal purchasing at four types of restaurant (Kim, 1989). Although there were significant patterns of use between the two groups in relation to the convenience foods, neither group was an overall heavier consumer of convenience foods. However, working wives showed significantly higher use than those not in paid employment of meal purchasing at all four types of restaurant and especially at two types, namely fast food and take-away restaurants (Kim, 1989).

Warde and Hetherington reported similar findings in their sample of UK households where 81% of women were in employment; take-away meals were purchased several times a week by 5% of households, weekly by 29% and monthly by 24% of households (Warde and Hetherington, 1994). However, unlike the North American studies cited above, Warde and Hetherington had no comparison group and it is difficult to draw conclusions from these findings.

The North American bias and more generally the lack of detail in the studies themselves makes it difficult to draw conclusions about potential for dietary change. The workplace has been targeted in the US as a venue for health promotional activities which have included a focus upon nutrition (US Department of Health and Human Service Public Health Service, 1993). This has also happened (although less often) in the UK, where there are some examples in the literature of 'healthy eating' interventions (for example, Sorenson *et al.*, 1990), although many are not published. The importance and potential of the workplace for studying nutritional issues related to women contrasts with the paucity of work in this field and more UK research is urgently required in this important area.

(ii) Pregnant women

The literature on pregnancy is concerned with lifestyle factors. The vast literature on smoking and drinking, in particular, relates primarily to the clinical outcome of pregnancy (Chalmers *et al.*, 1989). Likewise, there is a substantial consumer literature on experiences of motherhood (for example Oakley, 1980; Reid and Garcia, 1989) but in this literature questions about diet are seldom asked or raised by the mothers themselves. Despite this, what little work exists on the topic suggests that women see pregnancy as an opportunity for dietary change. The literature is methodologically homogeneous, being mainly composed of small-scale surveys carried out at a local level (Doyle *et al.*, 1982; Eiser and Eiser, 1985) although two more robust studies exist (Schofield, Wheeler and Stewart, 1987; Anderson, Campbell and Shepherd, 1993).

Pre-pregnancy

Barker's work highlighted the importance of the mother's diet before pregnancy upon the foetus (Barker, 1994) (see also Wynn *et al.*, 1994) and, although his work has its critics (Lucas, 1994), considerable interest has been expressed by members of the medical profession in the period of pre-pregnancy (for example Levitt, 1993; Cefalo, Bowes and Moos, 1995). While the importance of pre-conceptual care has been stressed in the medical literature for over a decade the notion of targeting women at this time has been criticised, for example by Lumley and Astbury (1989), and little empirical work has explored the awareness and understanding of pre-pregnancy for health professionals and consumers.

It appears to be accepted that pre-pregnant women and women in early pregnancy, should have access to vitamin supplementation. An MRC trial showed clear protective effects against neural tube defects for the group who took folic acid throughout pregnancy (MRC Vitamin Study Research Group, 1991). This study paved the way for the Department of Health's 1992 recommendations on folic acid, particularly folic acid intake during the preconceptual period and during early pregnancy. However, preconception clinics reportedly have different roles (for example Cox *et al.*, 1992; Pearson *et al.*, 1996), although all seem to recognise the importance of diet and vitamin supplementation in particular as essential features of the pre-conceptual period.

Within the remit of this review only one nutrition study was located which had pre-pregnancy as a key word, in which knowledge about diet was related to pre-pregnancy (Pearson *et al.*, 1996). These authors reported the findings from a questionnaire study of staff and clients at a family planning clinic in the UK. The medical and nursing staff of the clinic scored highly on nutritional questions about pregnancy, with a mean score of 91.8%, while clients (with a sample heavily biased towards teenagers) achieved a mean score of 77.6% (Pearson *et al.*, 1996). On the topic of folate supplementation 69% of staff and 12% of clients correctly responded to the question about the need for folate supplementation, while the authors noted that only one-quarter of the staff could state the correct dosage and none of the professional sample mentioned the need for a folate-rich diet. Clients scored lower, with an average of 34.3% on pregnancy-related topics (Pearson *et al.*, 1996).

The study is interesting in that it provides information about the knowledge level of professionals and non-pregnant women about pregnancy nutritional issues. Both groups had good general knowledge but both were less knowledgeable about the pregnancy specific questions (although little detail was provided in the publication about wording and level of complexity of the questions). The client sample was not drawn from women planning to become pregnant in the near future. The lack of knowledge from both medical and nursing staff does suggest that this is an area in which training may be appropriate. Whether folate supplementation comes under the pre-pregnancy or pregnancy heading it is important that professional staff have accurate knowledge.

Dietary changes

Real changes in women's diet are reported in the literature relating to pregnant women (for example Anderson *et al.*, 1993), suggesting that they are receptive to advice at this time but more research is needed on the nature and the emphasis of the advice. Knowledge is not sufficient to create change.

In a comparative study of pregnant women in England and Scotland, with 265 women sampled from antenatal clinics in London and Edinburgh hospitals (Schofield, Wheeler and Stewart, 1987; Stewart, Wheeler and Schofield, 1988; Schofield, Stewart and Wheeler, 1989), the researchers used a variety of methods including dietary records and interviews to study regional and social class differences in diet (Schofield, Wheeler and Stewart, 1987). Social class variations in dietary change were found but these were not in a consistent direction. Regarding mean energy intakes, few differences were detected between social classes, with no significant differences in the intake of protein, fat or fibre between women living in London and Edinburgh (Schofield, Wheeler and Stewart, 1988). Overall 58% Scots and 67% English women said that they had made voluntary changes to their diet (Stewart, Wheeler and Schofield, 1988).

Anderson and her colleagues studied pregnant and non-pregnant women's dietary behaviour and concluded likewise that 'pregnant women do eat differently from non-pregnant women'. They summarised these differences as consisting of less alcohol, a high nutrient density of protein and sodium and greater intakes of some minerals (Anderson, Campbell and Shepherd, 1993). Very similar findings were obtained from the small study by Eiser and Eiser (1985).

Waterson and Murray-Lyon studied smoking and drinking patterns of a large cohort of pregnant women attending a London antenatal clinic (Waterson and Murray-Lyon, 1989). When the researchers compared pre-pregnancy and pregnancy drinking levels they found that 42% of those who drank before they became pregnant reduced their alcohol consumption by the first trimester, the proportion of which increased to 60% by the third trimester (Waterson and Murray-Lyon, 1989).

Smoking has a more complicated relationship with diet and pregnancy, partly because of the overlap of smoking with a range of other social factors which themselves are thought to have a deleterious effect on pregnancy. Therefore the finding that smokers report different diets (for example Haste *et al.*, 1990; Trygg *et al.*, 1995) is difficult to interpret in itself. However, in Anderson's Scottish study smoking exerted an independent effect on intakes of protein, dietary fibre and vitamin C. In her study, smoking was the only factor affecting vitamin C intake, accounting for 10% of the variation (Anderson, 1991).

Pregnancy and material deprivation

In relation to 'access' issues, what little research there is on pregnant women living in material deprivation, suggests that their dietary concerns are similar to those of non-pregnant women (Doyle *et al.*, 1982; NCH, 1991), with research underlining the point that these women do not have the opportunity of their more well-off counterparts to change their diet. Thus in a study which sampled women attending a Salvation Army Mothers Hospital in London (Doyle *et al.*, 1982) the authors noted that 'energy levels of the sample were disturbingly low', with only 6% within RDAs for any one trimester while 71% of the sample were below RDAs for folate.

Knowledge, culture and attitudes

Purchasing and preparing foods has been shown to be influenced by food availability and cost, on the one hand, and by 'knowledge, culture and attitudes' towards specific foods on the other. The latter group of influences is far more difficult to analyse in terms of individual factors, and perhaps because of this, a number of studies simply use the shorthand 'culture' without elaborating upon which aspects of culture may be the most influential.

Access also links with culture and the connection between access and culture is recognised in policy documents, for example, in the sections on retail sector and community action in the Scottish Office document *Scotland's health, a challenge to us all. Eating for health: a diet action plan for Scotland* (Scottish Office, 1996). Thus, the restricted intake of fresh vegetables in the Scottish diet is partly due to (especially in the past) the restricted growth of certain types of vegetables (especially green leafy vegetables) which in turn means that common Scottish dishes do not include green vegetables or salads. A few studies have compared regional diets. For example, the Scottish diet has been compared with the English diet (Schofield, Wheeler and Stewart, 1987).

This is a diverse field of work, with a number of attitudinal studies being balanced by some good qualitative work which elaborates on the importance of nutritional issues for women.

Professional advice – women of childbearing age

The impact of professional advice is raised as a research topic more often when women undertake a caring role (for example pregnancy and looking after infants, see below) while few studies have looked at health professionals and advice giving to women of childbearing age. Murray and her colleagues surveyed 58 primary health professionals in Grampian, Scotland about their dietetic knowledge, a sample which included general practitioners, and community and practice nurses (Murray *et al.*, 1993). Asked about sources of nutritional information, only 14% ranked in-service training as important. Seventy-four per cent responded that they had never attended an in-service event or display on healthy eating. Respondents had a broad general knowledge about dietary factors (for example high fibre, low fat) but were more likely to be inaccurate over specific issues, with no significant variation between the different occupational groups. Knowledge about the roles of cholesterol and carbohydrates was limited and the authors highlight a lack of understanding about the ways in which different components of the diet interact (Murray *et al.*, 1993). The study findings suggest more training in nutritional issues is needed for these key professional groups.

Sociological studies of family eating patterns have taken a rather different approach and, often using qualitative methods, have focused upon the domestic relations within the family with relatively little reported about the impact of professional advice on dietary change. Calnan noted evidence from his small interview study that there were 'hints of scepticism' about food messages, the hints being stronger from working-class women (Calnan, 1990). In this study, not only did women have problems differentiating what constituted good advice but they also had limited scope for being able to put good advice into practice when they were constrained by limited resources and family preferences (Calnan, 1990), a finding supported by Mackie, Wood and Gregory (1993).

The HEA study of women on low income also reported conflict between the professional advice on diet and women's own priorities, summarising the findings by noting 'the less the money, the lower the morale and the shorter the perspective on health' (HEA, 1989, p. 13). However, the authors note that not all professional advice was seen by their sample as contradictory or irrelevant; the 'reduce fat, increase fibre' message was seen as plausible and important, and some women had attempted to reduce the amount of fat in their diet and had tried grilling rather than frying food (HEA, 1989).

Professional advice – pregnant women

Research is not extensive and findings are not conclusive as to the extent to which pregnant women attend to professional advice. Researchers have shown that many women are receptive to professional advice in pregnancy and do use health professionals as key sources of advice in pregnancy (Eiser and Eiser, 1985; Anderson, Campbell and Shepherd, 1993; Strychar, Griffiths and Conry, 1990). Although not the focus of the study, Charles and Kerr noted that the antenatal and child health clinics were the two venues where women were most likely to encounter professionals. Women in their sample commented unfavourably upon the nature of the advice, reporting that it was seen as inadequate and not related to the concerns women experienced in feeding a family (Charles and Kerr, 1988). Professional advice focused upon weight watching in pregnancy but the women were not given specific information about how to do this and what foods to be wary of in pregnancy (Charles and Kerr, 1988) (see also Best, Little and MacPherson, 1989). Kogan, in a large-scale retrospective US study of 9924 women, found that women were more likely to recall having received professional advice on taking vitamins and eating proper foods if they had more education, higher incomes and were married (Kogan *et al.*, 1994). This suggests that certain groups are more receptive to professional messages. Overall, these studies do not provide much information about the influence of the professional with dietary advice during pregnancy, but the increased frequency of contact suggests that this is a period of opportunity for professionals, even though at present the nature of the advice is not always seen as helpful.

Studies of professional advice and women's folate intake

A small number of studies report on knowledge of vitamin supplements, including folic acid, among women and professional staff (Best, Little and MacPherson, 1989; Mulliner, Spiby and Fraser, 1995) (see also the pre-pregnancy study of Pearson *et al.*, 1996, reported above). Three studies, carried out prior to the Department of Health's 1992 recommendations on folic acid, provide 'baseline' information on the topic of vitamin supplementation (Eiser and Eiser, 1985; Schofield, Stewart and Wheeler, 1989; Best, Little and MacPherson, 1989). Eiser and Eiser, in a small-scale study, asked women, who were between 12 and 16 weeks pregnant, about their knowledge of vitamin supplements during pregnancy. The authors report that 72.9% of women were already taking iron tablets, 16.7% did not know why iron was prescribed and 14.6% were taking vitamin supplements (Eiser and Eiser, 1985).

As part of their larger study, Schofield and her colleagues simply note that there were clear social class differences in their English/Scottish comparative study, with women from social classes I and II having higher mean intakes of folic acid (Schofield, Stewart and Wheeler, 1989).

In one further study (Best, Little and MacPherson, 1989), the researchers surveyed a sample of 246 pregnant women in an antenatal clinic, to ascertain the extent and determinants of vitamin supplementation in early pregnancy. The researchers found that about a quarter of the sample (23%) had taken the supplements for at least six months before they were pregnant, 17% started taking them when considering becoming pregnant, 19% when pregnant and 35% after their first visit to their general practitioner (Best, Little and MacPherson, 1989). About half the pregnant women in the study reported by Best and colleagues had discussed diet and specifically vitamin supplementation with others (a friend or relative) and about the same proportion of the sample had such a discussion with health professionals. Inconsistency in general practitioner advice was reported, some doctors suggesting that women take supplements, others that they did not (Best, Little and MacPherson, 1989). However, it is important to note that a relatively small proportion (15%) of the sample was drawn from early pregnancy, since the researchers recruited women from all three trimesters, not standardising for gestation.

Despite the Department of Health recommendations on folate (Expert Advisory Group, 1992), the limited research on the topic suggests that, five years on, these recommendations are not necessarily clearly understood. One study, carried out after the government had made these recommendations, has shown that a proportion of women still remain unaware of the significance of folate, particularly before conception, although the proportion of women who are aware rises once they know that they are pregnant. Clark and Fisk found a very small proportion (3%) of the 411 women they studied had taken folate before conception, while a further 2% had altered their diets to increase their intake of folate rich foods. Once pregnant, 26% of women increased their folate intake, 20% through tablets and 6% through diet, with only one woman doing both (Clark and Fisk, 1994).

Mulliner, Spiby and Fraser found, in a sample of 77 midwives in the Trent region, that 66% had received less than two hours training about nutrition during their training and 46% scored poorly in the knowledge section of the questionnaire. The largest proportion of midwives (48%) reported that they had gained their knowledge of nutritional issues from the media. Two-thirds indicated that they were anxious about their level of knowledge about specific nutritional issues (for example about vegetarian mothers and mothers with particular disease conditions) and about pre-conceptual nutritional and vitamin advice (Mulliner, Spiby and Fraser, 1995). This is a small sample and, without seeing the nutritional issues on which the midwives scored poorly, it is difficult to comment on the level of professional knowledge. However, that a large proportion of professionals was worried about the limitations of their knowledge suggests that there is a potential for more training among those groups which have high contact with women.

Overall, the lack of work in this area suggests that, in the first instance, more work is needed to find out in more detail women's knowledge and information channels on this topic. Both the study by Mulliner and colleagues and that by Clarke and Fisk suggest that professionals play a key role in helping women to understand the importance of early folate intake and to offer clear advice to women at this stage in the life cycle.

Attitudes toward eating and eating habits/food knowledge in women of childbearing age

Knowledge about diet has been explored in a number of studies ranging from very large-scale surveys to small-scale qualitative work (for example Cotunga *et al.*, 1992; Devine and Olson, 1992; Backett, 1992). Researchers carrying out qualitative work have been more sensitive to possible bias and have emphasised that studies focusing upon diet and dietary changes are not 'neutral' topics for respondents, many of whom may second-guess the more socially acceptable answers (Mayall, 1986; Backett, 1992). Mayall notes, for example, that she suspected that 'something that may have affected mothers' replies was that the interview was mainly about promoting health and preventing illness' (Mayall, 1986, p.98), the perceived focus of the study thus affecting the mothers' responses. Despite this methodological drawback, there are some clear messages from the existing research which are discussed below.

Several Scottish studies (Schofield, Wheeler and Stewart, 1988; Anderson, Campbell and Shepherd, 1993) have noted that confusion exists among many women about the respective roles of fibre, fats and carbohydrates. However, large-scale surveys in the US and the UK (Cotunga *et al.*, 1992; Blaxter, 1990), as well as smaller-scale interview studies (NCH, 1991; Backett, 1990), have indicated that many women have considerable knowledge about the foods which might be included in a healthy diet.

From the very detailed findings of the US 1987 National Health Interview Survey which, in one section, focused upon the links between disease and diet, 35.3% respondents (of both sexes) said that they had changed their diet within the past five years, with more reporting eating vegetables, low-fat meats and fruit (Cotunga *et al.*, 1992). Among the remaining 64.6% of respondents who said that they had *not* changed their diets, the most frequently cited reason was that they enjoyed the foods that they were eating (Cotunga *et al.*, 1992). A large percentage of this group (69.3%) said that they thought their diet was already 'healthful' (a response which tended to increase with age yet decrease with increasing income and educational level). Forty-eight per cent of the non-'changers' reported that the number of recommendations made it difficult to know which ones to follow (Cotunga *et al.*, 1992).

Blaxter and her colleagues carried out a Health and Lifestyle Survey with a national sample of 9003 men and women within the UK, with 3749 women between the ages of 18 and 59, i.e. within the age group of this review (Blaxter, 1990). The study yielded many relevant findings, some on regional variations reported above (Whichelow, Erzinclioglu and Cox, 1991). Blaxter found that when women were asked about why individuals may be healthier today, women placed more importance on food and diet and on standard of living, whereas men emphasised medicine and exercise (Blaxter, 1990).

The NCH study concluded from questionnaires and interviews with low-income families that 'there was no evidence to suggest that parents are ignorant about what constitutes a healthy diet' (NCH, 1991, p. 3) although, as already discussed, material constraints may affect the final decisions about food purchasing (NCH, 1991) (see also Dowler and Calvert, 1995). The HEA study likewise found that 'healthiness' of food was pushed down the list of priorities where women were constrained by resources (HEA, 1989).

Other studies from the US and the UK have taken a qualitative approach, with more middle-class samples. Such work includes Devine and Olson's study of a New York sample of 36 women who were interviewed about personal nutrition care (Devine and Olson, 1992), Backett's Edinburgh-based research (Backett, 1990) and Mayall's research on 135 mothers of varied social class (Mayall, 1986). All found that women were reflective when discussing their family's eating habits and took the issue of what they and their family ate seriously. When asked to comment on factors which affected health, diet was often rated highly as an important factor in sustaining good health (Mayall, 1986; Pill and Parry, 1989; Calnan, 1990). Mayall reports that class differences were evident in the ways in which diet (i.e. nutritional intake) was discussed. All but two mothers in her sample talked about food being of central importance for promoting optimal health and preventing ill health. There was, however, a steady drop in the number of times food was mentioned in connection with illness prevention and health promotion from social class I to classes IV and V (Mayall, 1986). In interpreting these results it is important that Mayall's reservations about possible bias are borne in mind.

Backett, as part of a two-year qualitative study with repeat interviews with a sample of middle-class Edinburgh families, investigated the relationship between health knowledge and behaviour. Backett noted the pressure for respondents to report biomedically determined knowledge about 'healthy lifestyles', with other kinds of health knowledge being expressed or given greater legitimacy in later interviews. The researcher commented that it was clear that knowledge is not always translated into behavioural practices, even in a health-promoting environment (Backett, 1992). This finding is evident in a number of other studies using a more structured approach (Parraga, 1990; Anderson, Campbell and Shepherd, 1995).

A number of studies have also emphasised the gulf between individuals' perception of what they ate (i.e. what they thought they ate) and what they reported eating (for example Backett, 1992; Anderson *et al.*, 1994a). Backett, for example, noted the discrepancy between individuals' accounts of what they 'typically' ate and the more detailed descriptions of their daily meals obtained in later interviews (Backett, 1992). Calnan noted that the difference between beliefs and actual consumption was more marked for working-class women in his small sample (Calnan, 1990). Research, therefore, suggests a clear opportunity in that many respondents are knowledgeable about what may constitute a 'good diet'. However, knowledge about diet does not necessarily lead to the consumption of a balanced diet. Other factors such as material deprivation and the preferences of all family members (see below) also influence the final decision.

The family influence on meal choice

Researchers investigating family meals (Graham, 1984; Backett, 1990; Mackie, Wood and Gregory, 1993) have noted that food choices tend to privilege the male partner and children, with women's food preferences being the least influential. Several studies have reported the more conservative approach of men (and children) to food choices (Charles and Kerr, 1988; Pill and Parry, 1989; Mackie, Wood and Gregory, 1993; Dowler and Calvert, 1995). Using focus groups, Mackie and her colleagues, found that their female respondents experienced conflicts in trying to produce a diet which conformed to their concept of being healthy (their term) but which also would be eaten by other family members (Mackie, Wood and Gregory, 1993). Pill and Parry's qualitative study in South Wales (Pill and Parry, 1989) found that support for positive health behaviours came from close family members, including husbands and children. The researchers found that women in their sample joined in with their partners' dietary changes. However, if a husband blocked his wife's efforts to diet then the woman often reverted to her original eating patterns or made separate meals. More generally they noted that while the researchers asked the (female) respondents about personal behaviour changes, the respondents responded with information about general family behaviours and changes (Pill and Parry, 1989).

A qualitative study from the US with 36 well-educated, middle to upper income women in New York echoes these findings. Devine and Olson analysed the interviews by focusing upon how women's social roles promoted or constrained nutritional care. The researchers found that women with young children attempted to play a number of positive roles, such as 'caretaker role', or 'teacher role', in relation to nutrition. However, women also devised strategies to deal with conflict between looking after their own nutritional needs and those of others (Devine and Olson, 1992). The 'peacekeeper role' involved the prevention of family conflicts at mealtimes and the respondents reported considerable family conflicts between the different wishes of the partner, the children and the mother regarding the types of food that were served (Devine and Olson, 1992).

These studies are helpful in that they identify the barriers which women face when attempting personal and family dietary change. Although women may carry out most of the meal preparation, and possibly even the shopping (to refer back to studies discussed above), decisions about actual foods consumed are affected by material factors, access to foods and, as the research discussed above has noted in particular, by the preferences and tastes of all family members. Thus an awareness of the significance of male and children's preferences is important when planning dietary change. This issue is returned to later in the review.

Styles of eating – eating out and snacking

Despite the reported trend towards increased consumption of food prepared and eaten outside the home (for example MAFF, 1995), there are few studies of the social context or the decision-making surrounding this choice, and little research on which to base comment on the impact of the trend upon women of childbearing age. An increasing percentage of the household food budget is devoted to 'eating out', rising from 9.8% in 1959–61 to 20.4% in 1991 (Martens and Warde, 1997). Martens and

Warde interviewed the principal food provider in 30 households 'diverse in their circumstances', and asked the interviewee *inter alia*, about attitudes to, and frequency of, eating out; they also interviewed 1001 individuals in three cities in England (Martens and Warde, 1997). Although their work will be published after the cut-off date for the review, data have been presented at conferences and some preliminary findings are included in this review.

The authors report a range of reasons why individuals liked to eat out which emphasised not only the venue itself but also the understandings and interpretations of the participants; thus the authors highlight variations in terms of expectations about the venue, different criteria of judgement and different reactions to food, service and decor (Martens and Warde, forthcoming). The authors have also explored other issues concerning everyday consumption and choices about 'eating out' and 'eating in' and gender issues to do with eating out (Martens, personal communication). The unusual focus of their research, exploring as it does the factors associated with 'social' eating out emphasises how little is known about the patterns of public food consumption.

Beardsworth and Keil, in one of the few research studies on the topic of vegetarianism, carried out a qualitative study using a snowball sample of 76 vegetarians and vegans (Beardsworth and Keil, 1993). They report that their respondents noted two ways in which vegetarian food was becoming incorporated into the mainstream retail food system. The first 'trend' was towards the greater availability of foodstuffs which made the preparation of vegetarian foods at home easier, and the second was the greater availability of vegetarian options when eating out (Beardsworth and Keil, 1993).

There is relatively little research on 'snacking' as a distinct form of food consumption, although this has been studied by a small number of researchers. Story, in the US, studied adolescents and snacking behaviour (Story, 1989). Anderson *et al.* included questions on snacking in the West of Scotland Twenty-07 study (Anderson, Macintyre and West, 1993). In addition, snacking is mentioned in a few of the qualitative studies of family eating habits included in this review (for example Mayall, 1986; Charles and Kerr, 1988).

The Health and Lifestyle Survey found a far higher proportion of British adults in the 18–29 age group consumed one or two snacks a day than the older age groups (Cox *et al.*, 1987); other studies have focused upon the younger age groups. Story's US study of adolescent snacking behaviour (both sexes) suggests that food practices reported in the study are 'accentuated in adolescence' but are in fact typical of the American population and include 'diets high in sugar, saturated fats and sodium, missed meals, eating on the run, being too busy to eat, reliance upon convenience and fast foods, dieting and fad dieting' (Story, 1989). The American study noted that time was an important issue for the adolescents whom they studied and that various issues related to time were used to justify snacking (for example inconvenience of eating properly, too busy to worry about meals, too much trouble and expense to prepare healthy meals) (Story and Resnick, 1986).

Snacking in itself is not nutritionally unsound. However the nature of the snack is highly influenced by culture, and culturally acceptable snacks are defined very precisely as consisting of particular foods. Thus in the West of Scotland Twenty-07 study the adolescent sample (aged 15, men and women) reported 'grazing'. They recorded an average of 5.5 eating occasions per day, 2.7 of which were main meals while 2.8 were snacks (Anderson, Macintyre and West, 1993). The proportions of the adolescent sample which reported eating meals that included specific items at least once per day were as follows: chips (15%), crisps (43%), soft drinks (52%), sweets and/or chocolates (42%) (Anderson, Macintyre and West, 1993). The majority of foods consumed by the adolescents in Story's research were what they termed junk foods, including burgers, pizzas, chips and other fast foods, and foods which were notably high in fat and/or sugar (Story, 1989).

Charles and Kerr's female respondents reported that if men were left to feed the family they were more likely to provide 'snacks', which implied less cooking. The women also said that they consumed snacks between meals. These were more often biscuits and sweets rather than fruit (Charles and Kerr, 1988). Some suggested that a lunchtime 'snack' was acceptable but the use of convenience foods instead of a properly cooked main meal was less acceptable and more guilt-inducing (Charles and Kerr, 1988). If snacking is a form of food consumption that is popular, then the potential for dietary change should be recognised. At present it appears that snacking involves less nutritious groups of foods. Snacks will be further discussed in the section on children aged 1–5, but clearly it is an important topic worthy of more research attention.

Vegetarians

Vegetarians have been increasing in number in UK households. Recent polls suggest that a growing number of households contain a vegetarian member (Gallup Poll for the *Daily Telegraph*, April 1996; NOP survey for Hill and Knowlton/Tesco, 1996). The polls also suggest a cluster of social characteristics related to vegetarianism with non-meat eaters being more likely to be middle class and having completed their education after the age of 19 (RSL Nutritional Labelling Study for MAFF, 1995). There is reportedly a greater proportion of vegetarians who are women than men (see below) but the term 'vegetarian' itself has a number of definitions (see annex IV, Department of Health, 1994) which has resulted in non-comparable studies reporting on groups with different dietary patterns. Thus Santos and Booth report that more of their sample of 158 non-meat eaters were women (although the sample was one of convenience selected from those who chose a vegetarian dish at a university refectory). The majority of women reported eating vegetarian meals both at university and home (Santos and Booth, 1996). However, the overall sample contained a proportion who avoided only certain meats and it is difficult to draw further conclusions from their findings.

Hamilton (1993) studied attitudes towards 'wholefoods and health foods' in two different English populations. The first group comprised a cross-section of 304 members of the public (with a bias towards those with 'alternative' lifestyles) and the second group, a non-random sample of consumers with an 'alternative' lifestyle gathered from individuals attending an alternative festival near London. Hamilton found a cluster of beliefs and attitudes with, for example, a strong relationship between vegetarianism and alternative therapies (Hamilton, 1993). Of the festival sample, 74% followed unorthodox diets and 60% reported being vegetarian, and in both groups Hamilton found (as did Santos and Booth, 1996) that a higher proportion of women than men were following a vegetarian or 'whole, health or organic' diet. Hamilton notes that females in the younger age groups (between 16 and 35) showed a particularly high rate of vegetarianism (Hamilton, 1993).

Beardsworth and Keil carried out an interview study with 76 self-reported vegetarians; their findings show that whatever the motives of individuals becoming vegetarian, health was given high priority (Beardsworth and Keil, 1991). This review cannot discuss the nutritional merits or otherwise of vegetarian diets. Nevertheless, given this particular trend, it would be helpful to have more research on the topic, for example, examining the decision-making surrounding the change to a vegetarian diet and investigating how families adapt to this particular food preference.

Fruit and vegetable consumption

Increasing interest in the role that fruit and vegetables may play in protecting against CHD, cardiovascular disease and certain cancers has led to public campaigns to encourage more intake of these foods (Scottish Office, 1996). The topic of fruit and vegetables has been the focus of a number of research projects using a variety of methods, from large-scale telephone surveys (for example Serdula *et al.*, 1995) to smaller, qualitative studies (Kilcast, Cathro and Morris, 1996). Nutrition and Food Science (1996) reported on a number of MAFF-funded studies (for example see Kilcast, Cathro and Morris, 1996) with several focusing upon attitudes towards fruit and vegetables. Articles in the printed media (for example *Glasgow Herald*, 22 January 1997) have also reported innovative ways of introducing vegetables into the diet.

Large-scale surveys in the US and the UK confirm that women report a higher level of fruit and vegetable consumption than men do (Serdula *et al.*, 1995; MAFF, 1995). The short telephone survey of 23 699 adults in 16 US states confirmed that a higher proportion of women than men reported consuming five or more fruits or vegetables per day (22.6% compared with 17.5% for men) and that women were more likely than men to consume fruit (Serdula *et al.*, 1995). These findings are congruent with those of another US study (Dittus, Hilliers and Beerman, 1995) in which over a 1000 adults in Washington State were surveyed about attitudes to, and consumption of, fruit and vegetables. Dittus and her colleagues report that men had significantly higher scores than women based on attitudinal statements about barriers to fruit and vegetable intake.

Calnan, in a UK qualitative study which comments specifically upon fruit and vegetable consumption, found that individuals from his sample spoke about fruit and vegetables as (morally) 'good' and 'healthy' foods (Calnan, 1990) while Mackie and her colleagues also found that certain vegetables had a particular cultural image, with salads not being seen as 'manly food' (Mackie, Wood and Gregory, 1993). Cox and his colleagues studied adults' beliefs about fruit, vegetables and vegetable dishes and report that respondents scored taste, healthful, nutritious, family liking and fitting into eating habits as the top five beliefs for fruit, vegetables and vegetable dishes; however, in all assessments (for example intention to increase consumption) vegetable dishes came out lowest of the three foods (Cox *et al.*, 1996).

Studies of family meals (for example Murcott, 1983; Mayall, 1986) provide evidence on the 'cultural' role of vegetables. Murcott, in her anthropological study of 37 expectant mothers in South Wales (Murcott, 1983) was one of the first researchers to focus upon the importance of 'a proper meal' for women. Such meals included vegetables as an integral component. Mayall, too, noted that vegetables are highly valued as part of a main course. She observed, 'It is a commonplace idea that people consider a good main meal consists of meat and two vegetables' (Mayall, 1986, p. 101). Eighty-nine per cent of her sample made statements which agreed with this viewpoint.

Anderson *et al.* (1994a) and Cox *et al.* (1996) cite cost, lack of will-power, poor motivation and family influences as reasons given for the low intake of fruit and vegetables. Both these studies report that one problem is that many people (genders not differentiated) felt that their own intake of fruit and vegetables was higher than other people's, even when they had objectively scored 'low' on the intake scale (Anderson *et al.*, 1994a; Cox *et al.*, 1996).

It is evident from national surveys (Gregory *et al.*, 1990), as well as smaller-scale research (Anderson, Macintyre and West, 1993), that potatoes have a special status among vegetables, being consumed as snacks (crisps and chips) in considerable quantities. Anderson and her colleagues found that, while Scottish men and women do not eat large quantities of vegetables (see Scottish Office, 1993), potatoes, especially if fried, were acceptable. Looking at adolescent eating habits (men and women not differentiated) in the West of Scotland this same study revealed the heavy consumption of chips every day, and that these were eaten with other high fat foods (Anderson, Macintyre and West, 1994), while an earlier study (Cresswell *et al.*, 1983) cited in Anderson's study reported that chips were never served with (other) vegetables. In another study of adult eating patterns, Anderson and her colleagues also found that less than 4% of the adult sample were meeting or exceeding the WHO recommendations of at least 400 g of fruit and vegetables per day and more than 50% of all subgroups studied were eating less than half this recommended amount (Anderson *et al.*, 1994b).

The West of Scotland survey of fruit and vegetable eating with two cohorts of adults (Anderson *et al.*, 1994b) confirms the importance of studying overall eating patterns rather than isolating the consumption of particular foods. Anderson and her colleagues found correlations between fruit and vegetable consumption and certain 'main meal' items, for example a positive correlation (of fruit and vegetables) with chicken and a negative correlation with sausages and pies (Anderson *et al.*, 1994b).

The above research is not specifically confined to women and indeed often does not analyse the responses by gender. It may be that men and women have rather different beliefs and attitudes towards vegetables. What is clear, however, is that quite fine distinctions are made between different vegetables and different forms of cooking and presentation of these vegetables. The findings are, too, somewhat contradictory, with the qualitative work emphasising the relevance of vegetables to particular meals (an opportunity) while other research has tended to emphasise the restrictiveness of consumption of certain vegetables (a barrier).

Kilcast, Cathro and Morris (1996) present further evidence about vegetable purchasing and eating. The researchers carried out in-depth interviews followed by group discussions in four centres (English and Scottish) as the first part of an intervention study. Reporting on the consumer research, they distinguished 'high vegetable users' from 'low vegetable users'. The 'high vegetable users' were more 'active' in their attitudes and possessed a series of characteristics, showing a high level of control over the family members and eating patterns with a considerable advance planning of menus. High vegetable users held an experimental approach to eating, a strong food focus as part of their lifestyle and high self-esteem regarding family eating habits. By contrast, the low vegetable users were more passive, more likely to react to requests from the family (particularly the children), routine purchasing, strong lack of control over family feeding and family members eating different meals at different times (Kilcast, Cathro and Morris, 1996). The authors noted evidence from the low vegetable users of feelings of guilt about the family diet consistent with qualitative studies.

Studies of fruit and vegetable eating from other countries highlight the cultural shaping of attitudes towards these foods. Findings from a small study of low income families in Australia (Crotty, Rutishauser and Cahill, 1992) indicate that the expenditure and consumption of fruit and vegetables (cheap foods in Australia) was *higher* in the low-income families than in an average Australian household. Kilcast, Cathro and Morris (1996) cite MAFF surveys as indicating the relatively low consumption levels of fruit and vegetables compared to much of Europe, while regional variations within the UK have also been noted (for example Anderson, Macintyre and West, 1993). In a survey of a sample of West of Scotland adolescents from the Twenty-07 study, Anderson and her colleagues noted a contrast between the diet of Scottish school children and that of their French contemporaries. They noted the avoidance of salads and fresh leafy vegetables was more marked in the Scottish sample. The authors reported that 86% of the French school children ate green vegetables, 74% ate fresh fruit and 45% had fruit juice daily, in comparison to the Scottish adolescents who ate less than half these proportions (cited in Anderson, Macintyre and West, 1994).

These latter studies, as well as others reviewed above, start to unravel the complex set of beliefs and attitudes which are rather crudely classified as 'culture'; only when cultural beliefs can be understood can dietary change be attempted. High fruit and vegetable consumption tends to be combined with other social factors, such as class, education and 'lifestyle', as the studies by Kilcast, Cathro and Morris (1996), Anderson, Macintyre and West (1993) and Beardsworth and Keil (1991) have demonstrated. When investigating dietary change, then, it is important not to isolate and focus upon dietary change itself, but to understand that certain foods are associated with a broader set of cultural beliefs and behaviours.

Attitudes toward eating habits/food knowledge in pregnancy

Although pregnancy itself is an experience rich in cultural variation (Kitzinger, 1982), there is relatively little research on cultural practices and attitudes of pregnant women to diet and dietary change. No studies which focused specifically on attitudes to diet and pregnancy were located in the pre-pregnancy search; Anderson's study is perhaps closest. In a comparative study of pregnant and non-pregnant women, Anderson and her colleagues consecutively sampled 100 pregnant women visiting an Aberdeen antenatal clinic and a matched sample of 100 non-pregnant women. In terms of nutritional knowledge, there were no differences between the groups. The poorest score related to knowledge about carbohydrate. However, questions revealed significant differences in attitude and intention between the two groups. Behaviour belief items on coronary heart disease and maintaining health revealed a stronger relationship between these beliefs and intention to change to a healthier diet in pregnant women than in the non-pregnant. The correlation between maintaining health and intention was also significantly greater for pregnant women (Anderson, Campbell and Shepherd, 1993).

In the 'English/Scottish' comparative study of attitudes, Stewart and her colleagues attempted to explore social class and cultural influences on pregnant women's attitudes towards diet (Stewart, Wheeler and Schofield, 1988). In one publication, regional differences were highlighted, with the authors reporting that Scottish women had a more 'pragmatic' attitude towards food intake when pregnant, being less anxious than their English contemporaries, about their (physical) shape and less likely to eat recommended foods if they did not like them. Fewer Scots women reported that they wanted to know about diet when pregnant (36% of Scots, 63% English). Over half of both samples reported making 'voluntary' changes to their diet (Scots 58%, English 67%), with more from both groups (Scots 87%, English 93%) making 'involuntary' changes (craving and aversions) (differences not statistically significant). The authors report that a varying, though small, proportion of women reported on food they 'should' eat but which they avoided in practice because they disliked them (these included vegetables, liver and cheese) (Stewart, Wheeler and Schofield, 1988).

In a further analysis of this study, Stewart and her colleagues found that a proportion of women in both countries reported that they wanted to know about diet when they became pregnant, although regional and class differences were apparent with significantly more English women (63%) than Scots (36%) and more middle-class women (46% Scots, 77% English) than working-class (24% Scots, 47% English) women wanting to know (Stewart, Wheeler and Schofield, 1988). In a further discussion of pregnant women's knowledge of health issues, the researchers report that, when asked specific knowledge-based questions about fats, salt, dietary fibre, sugar and slimming, more London-based women responded correctly, with the lowest proportion of Scots women in manual social classes answering correctly (Schofield, Wheeler and Stewart, 1988).

Discussing the 'culture of pregnancy', Murcott examined women's views on dietary changes, particularly aversions and cravings, through interviews with a sample of 37 pregnant women living in South Wales (Murcott, 1988). Murcott argued that such dietary experiences were very personal, some reporting a range of changes during pregnancy, others emphasising the normality of pregnancy. There were, however, some common features, with fruit mentioned as a popular craving, and strong drinks (tea, coffee or alcohol) mentioned as a common aversion (Murcott, 1988).

These studies, combined with others already reviewed, confirm that pregnancy is not only a time of dietary change but that attitudes towards dietary change are very positive. However, knowledge about important dietary issues appears to take years to filter through and studies report uneven knowledge and uptake of government advice among both professionals and consumers.

3. Infants under 1 year

This section deals with literature relating to infant liquid and solid feeding. There are relatively few studies which focus on solid feeding for infants. However, there is evidence that the Department of Health recommendations in relation to solid feeding are not always being followed and, although some research deals with the issues rather superficially, there are pointers to where the key opportunities and barriers lie.

Although the move from infant liquid feeding to solid feeding occurs as a single process in life, the literature dealing with the nutritional intake of infants treats these two as quite distinct events. Few studies report on both liquid and solid feeding. The infant liquid feeding literature ('breast or bottle') is heavily quantitative with a number of randomised controlled trials (for example Frank *et al.*, 1987; Evans, Lyons and Killien, 1986). Because of the importance of the quantitative work in this area the review, exceptionally, draws upon these trials. Few researchers have chosen the qualitative approach (but see McIntosh, 1985; 1986), and thus the mothers' voices about their preferences are seldom heard directly.

Access

Although breastfeeding has long been viewed by experts as the nutritionally superior way to feed an infant (Department of Health and Social Security, 1988), it has not received such popularity with the general public. The majority of women in the UK fall short of breastfeeding for the optimum four-month period and data from the OPCS surveys on infant feeding in Great Britain confirm no changes in overall rate of breastfeeding over a ten-year period, with 63% mothers in 1990, compared with 65% in 1980, starting to breastfeed (White, Freeth and O'Brien, 1992). Research indicates that there are two main issues: a significant proportion of women (37%) choose not to breastfeed their child at all, while many do not continue breastfeeding for the recommended duration of four months. Although 63% of women start to breastfeed, only a minority, 39%, are still breastfeeding by 4 months and 33% by 6 months (White, Freeth and O'Brien, 1992).

Antenatal decision-making about infant feeding methods

In his Manchester survey, James found that the majority of mothers, whether they were breast or bottle feeding their infants, had decided upon feeding method before they became pregnant (James, 1981). This finding has been confirmed in subsequent studies (Holt and Wolkind, 1983; Hally *et al.*, 1984). Maehr and her colleagues found that in their sample of 96 teenage and 'adult' women (the latter being mothers aged between 23 and 33, matched to the teenage sample by ethnicity and date of delivery) from several ethnic groups, teenage mothers were less likely to make the decision about feeding method before pregnancy than were the 'adults' (Maehr *et al.*, 1993). There is some evidence which suggests that health professionals can influence the decision during the antenatal period (for example Hally *et al.*, 1984; Salt *et al.*, 1994).

Salt and colleagues contacted mothers in two English cities and interviewed them postnatally (Salt *et al.*, 1994). About half the mothers in both groups (51% in Salisbury, 41% in Durham) reported that during pregnancy they had been actively encouraged to breastfeed and that those who had been encouraged were more likely to breastfeed. Encouragement had mostly come from health visitors or midwives (43%, 32%) with other sources (husbands, mothers, friends) constituting only small percentages (Salt *et al.*, 1994).

Hospital practices

The most recent OPCS survey on infant feeding reveals that the steepest decline in breastfeeding comes in the first week after birth when 15% of mothers abandon the practice (12% having given up by the time they left hospital) (White, Freeth and O'Brien, 1992). In 1988, the Department of Health focused attention on hospital practices when it recommended practices which were felt to encourage breastfeeding, such as the early initiation of breastfeeding after the birth, 'rooming-in' and the avoidance of complementary feeds or fluids of any sort (Department of Health and Social Security, 1988). White and her colleagues report on several positive changes between 1980 and 1990 to hospital practices which favour breastfeeding, namely a decline in set feeding times, a considerable increase in the practice of keeping the baby at the bedside (from 17% in 1980 to 63% in 1990), and a decline in staff giving bottle feeds to breastfed infants (White, Freeth and O'Brien, 1992).

One important international influence in this field has been the Baby Friendly Hospitals Initiative (BFHI) which was jointly launched world-wide in 1991 by WHO and UNICEF and aimed at changing the hospital environment in order to improve breastfeeding rates. The initiative has directly and indirectly influenced a number of studies, including the US study of Wright, Rice and Wells, 1996, reported below. However, no research has been identified evaluating the impact of the initiative on UK mothers. Campbell and his colleagues report on an audit study in Fife which was designed to assess the success of the initiative in one hospital (Campbell, Gorman and Wigglesworth, 1995). There is a debate about the actual impact of the initiative as opposed to the intended, with anecdotal reports that staff are pressurising mothers to breastfeed against their will (Turner, 1996).

Breastfeeding interventions in hospital – intervention studies

A number of studies, using a variety of methods, have explored the impact of hospital practices upon infant feeding both in the UK and elsewhere. Interventions to encourage breastfeeding are numerous and the literature contains a number of intervention studies. Some are not clearly evaluated. For example, a number of peer counsellor programmes are being implemented in the UK, the evaluation of which is not published (Wright, 1996). Others have small samples and are aimed at culturally distant groups (for example Maehr *et al.*, 1993). There are nevertheless two randomised controlled trials (both carried out before the introduction of the BFHI) which deal specifically with hospital influences on breastfeeding (Jones and West, 1986; Carty and Bradley, 1990) and three other rigorous studies which are reviewed below.

To study the effectiveness of a lactation nurse, Jones and West, in their UK trial, randomised 678 women who breastfed at least once into an experimental group, in which mothers were attended by a lactation nurse, and a control group (Jones and West, 1986). The lactation nurse attended to practical problems as well as giving support and encouragement to women attempting to breastfeed. Women were interviewed 12 months after discharge to ascertain duration of breastfeeding, and after losses, this yielded a final sample of 393 women. The study found clear differences, with more of the experimental group (84%) than the control group (72%) still breastfeeding by 4 weeks and with benefit appearing greatest among social classes IV and V in these early weeks. There were consistent differences between the two groups up until 6 months (Jones and West, 1986). The published details of the trial lack sufficient statistical information to comment further on significance.

Carty and Bradley's Canadian trial focused upon the role of early discharge in influencing maternal and infant physical and psychological health, duration of breastfeeding and patient satisfaction, with a sample of 131 volunteers (Carty and Bradley, 1990). Women were randomised into three groups, two trials groups of varying discharge periods (12–24 hours, 25–48 hours) with a control group who underwent the traditional stay (4 days). In relation to breastfeeding, 87% in the early discharge groups and 79% in the traditional stay group were still breastfeeding after a month and, while the authors comment positively upon the length of breastfeeding of these groups, the differences were not statistically significant and the study contained a number of methodological problems (Carty and Bradley, 1990). Whether or not breastfeeding was maintained for 4–6 months is also not known.

A study by Bloom and colleagues used a less rigorous design when researching factors affecting feeding choice; the authors reported that breastfeeding mothers were 'randomly assigned' to an experimental or a control group while a group of formula feeding mothers became a third study group (Bloom *et al.*, 1982). The experimental group of mothers were given support for feeding by receiving three telephone calls at one-week intervals and provided with an information pamphlet. They found that the experimental and control group of breastfeeding mothers did vary in the duration of breastfeeding with the experimental group feeding for, on average, one week longer (Bloom *et al.*, 1982).

Two other studies have adopted a 'before-and-after' structure to the study of breastfeeding interventions. Using a variety of methods Winikoff and her colleagues studied the practices relating to breastfeeding in one hospital serving a low-income area in the US (Winikoff *et al.*, 1987). They found that more mothers were interested in breastfeeding than actually achieved it, while a staff survey revealed low morale about their ability to promote breastfeeding within this population.

Following a number of interventions in the hospital, which included staff in-service training, the introduction of a breastfeeding nurse/counsellor, educational materials and a telephone hot-line for mothers, the researchers evaluated the situation (Winikoff *et al.*, 1987). In this post-intervention study which included observation, interviews with staff and mothers, and chart reviews, the researchers reported an increase in mothers ever breastfeeding (i.e. at least once) from 15% to 56% at the end of the study period and a rise in exclusive breastfeeding ($^3/_4$ of all feedings) from 0% to 15% in the study hospital. This latter rate of exclusive breastfeeding compared favourably with that of a 'control' hospital where over the same time period the rate had increased only from 5% to 7% (Winikoff *et al.*, 1997). Because of the lack of proper controls in the design of the study and the varied nature of the interventions it is not possible to ascertain which aspect(s) of the interventions effected the changes and a full statistical analysis is not presented.

Wright and her colleagues report on a 'before-and-after' project which set out to improve feeding practices in a university hospital in Arizona (Wright, Rice and Wells, 1996). Explicitly influenced by the BFHI, the researchers carried out a baseline study in 1990 and subsequently introduced a range of policies and practices positively to encourage breastfeeding. The study was evaluated with a survey and follow-up telephone interviews. The number of women who breastfed within an hour of birth increased considerably (24.8% in 1990 to 63.2% in 1993) and the number reporting receiving help with breastfeeding also increased from 61.3% to 81.9%. Among the other findings was greater likelihood of mothers continuing to breastfeed to 4 months if they had been given the name of a support person or group (Wright, Rice and Wells, 1996).

It is clear that changes in hospital practices have been made (for example, by increasing the practice of rooming-in), with the explicit intention of promoting breastfeeding. One must set against these adjustments to hospital routines, however, evidence from national surveys which indicates that over the same time-frame there has been an almost stable rate in the uptake of breastfeeding. The intervention studies have attempted to measure the effect of changing hospital practices on breastfeeding rates in a structured manner; after reviewing the literature it appears that few studies are methodologically of high quality (or are well reported) and the findings are not clear-cut. The studies do suggest that some interventions are helpful in encouraging the change to breastfeeding, but the diversity of the research contexts does not allow us to report more.

Breastfeeding interventions in hospital – descriptive studies

Descriptive studies likewise provide ambiguous findings about the significance of hospital policies and staff. Wright and Walker (1983) and Reiff and Essock-Vitale (1985) studied infant feeding before the BFHI was proposed. Wright and Walker's survey of a large random sample of 617 first-time mothers underlined the importance of the early establishment of breastfeeding. One significant finding from their survey was that if the mother breastfed within 12 hours the likelihood was increased of sustaining that form of feeding (Wright and Walker 1983). However, the authors note that this association was complex, and was related to the mother's social class and education and was not significantly related to subsequent duration of feeding or feeding routines, among other factors.

Reiff and Essock-Vitale found, in their study of the influence of hospital practices on infant feeding choice, that the great majority of the 50 staff interviewed reported that they discussed infant feeding 'routinely or often' with mothers (92%) and 85% reported that they routinely counselled mothers to breastfeed. Eighty-one per cent of nursing staff felt that certain mothers should be encouraged to bottle feed, including those with infants who were ill, high risk, or premature, and mothers who had insufficient milk supply, breast or nipple problems and those stating a desire to bottle feed (Reiff and Essock-Vitale, 1985). In the same study only 54% of the consecutive sample of 77 mothers reported talking to the staff about infant feeding, and 68% of this group interpreted these discussions as advocating breastfeeding. The researchers also reported a substantial number of mothers changing from breast to bottle feeding during the first two weeks and concluded that 'non verbal teaching by modelling is more effective than verbal counselling in this regard' (Reiff and Essock-Vitale 1985, p.877).

In a more recent study following the BFHI, Beeken and Waterston's postal questionnaire to health workers (hospital and community midwives and health visitors) and mothers found variation in hospital practices intended to facilitated breastfeeding (Beeken and Waterston, 1992). Generally, however, staff responses suggested 'good practice'; for example most (85%) reported that rooming-in after, the first night was practised 'frequently' or 'very frequently' and 64% reported that breastfed babies were 'infrequently' given dextrose, glucose or top-up bottle feeds (Beeken and Waterston, 1992).

Bruce and colleagues studied influences on the take-up rate of breastfeeding in a sample of hospital staff and mothers at the same hospital (Bruce, Khan and Olsen, 1991). A sample of mothers were interviewed at two days postpartum and sent a postal questionnaire at six weeks, and data from a smaller sample of hospital staff were collected using a self-administered questionnaire. Of the staff sample (hospital and community midwives), 73% agreed that there should either be no policy on infant feeding or that it should be neutral, while 31% agreed that there was usually or always enough time to talk to mothers planning to breastfeed (Bruce *et al.*, 1991). In the six-week questionnaire the majority of women (79%) reported that they were 'satisfied' or 'very satisfied' with the hospital support and policy but 57% agreed that the advice they received about infant feeding from the staff was 'mostly' or 'partly' conflicting. About a third of the sample (35%) thought that staff took a neutral position and a half (49%) thought that breastfeeding was supported (Bruce, Khan and Olsen, 1991).

In the follow-up study (Bruce and Griffioen, 1995), subsequent to the introduction of a breastfeeding adviser in the unit, there was an increase in staff supporting the statement that the unit should have a policy on baby feeding, although the majority of staff still agreed with the 'neutral position' view (but numbers in this study were very small) (Bruce and Griffioen, 1995).

A number of studies report that a minority of staff in the maternity services were less enthusiastic about breastfeeding (for example hospital and community midwives) (Bruce and Griffioen, 1995; Beeken and Waterston, 1992). In Beeken and Waterston's Newcastle-based project the majority of health professionals agreed or strongly agreed 'that there is no need to wean a baby from the breast before 4 months' (83%); 'lay organisations should be more widely advertised' (71%); and 'breastfed babies are healthier babies' (65%) (Beeken and Waterston, 1992).

However, a significant minority of Beeken and Waterston's staff sample reported disagreeing with positive statements about breastfeeding (for example 47% disagreed or strongly disagreed that 'milk company advertising should be banned in antenatal clinics' and 28% disagreed that 'breastfed babies are healthier') (Beeken and Waterston, 1992). Bergman, in a Swedish study set up to study potential barriers to breastfeeding among staff at a variety of maternity settings, found that about half the staff considered their knowledge to be insufficient and they felt it was 'difficult' or 'rather difficult' to work with issues relating to breastfeeding (Bergman *et al.*, 1994). The study also reported the staff's concern about their work load vis-à-vis the perceived time needed to provide information on breastfeeding with 82% of staff experiencing their workload as 'heavy' or 'very heavy' (Bergman *et al.*, 1994).

In Becker's study in rural Ireland (Becker, 1992) where breastfeeding rates on discharge varied in the three study hospitals between 29% and 31% of mothers (1989 figures), the researcher found that midwives' knowledge of breastfeeding (indicated by agreement to statements) was quite poor with only 20% correctly answering nine questions asked in the questionnaire. When responses to a particular question were compared, however, about three-quarters of the responses from midwives were found to be consistent, with around three-quarters in agreement with each other (with poor agreement within the group of obstetricians and high agreement within the paediatricians, although there were small samples for these two latter groups) (Becker *et al.*, 1992).

Hospital practices are important influences and can constitute strong barriers or opportunities. Descriptive studies mirror intervention studies in failing to offer a clear picture. There is evidence of variation in practice between hospitals, and among staff in terms of their views towards breastfeeding. Changing hospital practices may be an easier task than changing the views of staff about infant feeding and it may be that more attention is required to be directed towards the latter task. Having more time to spend with the mothers and specific training regarding breastfeeding are issues suggested by this literature.

Work and breastfeeding

Although the mother's return to work is more likely to fall within the period of solid feeding of the infant (the vast majority of women do not continue breastfeeding beyond the first few months), research has concentrated on the impact of women's return to work upon sustained breastfeeding. Even here there are very few studies. The most recent

OPCS survey suggests a link between work and feeding. Fewer mothers (31%) who returned to work when their baby was aged between 6 weeks and 4 months were still breastfeeding at 4 months compared to 48% of similar mothers who did not go back to work until after the baby was 4 months old (White, Freeth and O'Brien, 1992). A Danish prospective study (Weile *et al.*, 1990) with a postal questionnaire sent monthly to the sample over the first year of the infant's life (overall response rate 72%) reported on the decline in breastfeeding among their sample of 548 mothers. The researchers found that the infant being placed in day care (used here as a proxy for mother's return to work) was a significant factor in breastfeeding cessation (Weile *et al.*, 1990).

One US study has been identified as falling within the remit of this review (Auerbach, 1984). Auerbach's study is not strong, using a volunteer sample from magazines, with 567 women from a variety of occupational backgrounds completing the questionnaire retrospectively at widely different time points. From a list of possible problems facing working mothers, 'fatigue' was ranked as the highest, followed by 'finding time at work to pump/express milk' and 'worry about milk supply' (two of these three concerns were also expressed by non-working mothers). Nearly half of employers (44%) were unaware of the fact that the women were breastfeeding. Eighty-two per cent of women said that they would breastfeed again (Auerbach, 1988).

Confounding factors in this kind of study are serious: the Auerbach study contains its own biases (volunteer sample, non-standardised retrospective survey) but the large-scale studies reviewed above have not included the workplace policies as significant explanatory factors. In the UK, too, it is very difficult to examine returning to work and breastfeeding status in isolation; women in professional occupations may have a more tolerant management, more flexible working hours and more workplace opportunities for breastfeeding than the majority of working women, while conditions of maternity leave may differ between occupations. Conversely, Morrow and Barraclough, citing other research, note that for some women the decision to return to work precludes breastfeeding, given the inflexible hours of many forms of employment for non-professional women (Morrow and Barraclough, 1993). In order to identify barriers and opportunities more accurately, stronger UK-based research is required to study the circumstances of women returning to a variety of working situations. Workplace policies and employers' attitudes are also highly relevant and warrant separate research.

Income and infant solid feeding

Although breastfeeding is essentially a free way to feed the infant (compared to the costs involved with buying formula and the related equipment), cost is very seldom mentioned in studies about liquid feeding choice. However, nearly one-fifth (17%) of women surveyed in the most recent OPCS survey reported planning to breastfeed because it was cheaper than bottle-feeding (White, Freeth and O'Brien, 1992). As soon as the infant progresses beyond that stage, family income has a stronger influence on feeding decisions. A series of randomised controlled trials evaluating the impact of free gift packs of dried milk and other related items from commercial companies form a significant contribution to the field.

In a follow-up study to a randomised controlled trial of social support in pregnancy, Oakley and Rajan sent out detailed questionnaires to the participating mothers one year after the birth of their infant (Oakley and Rajan, 1993). Oakley and Rajan found a strong social class difference in the amount of protein given to the baby in the previous twenty-four hours; mothers living on low income were significantly more likely to give their infant fewer foods containing meat, fish, cheese or egg. Likewise they report that middle-class mothers were more likely to give their infants more fresh fruit, salad and leafy vegetables than working class mothers (Oakley and Rajan, 1993).

Iron is an important component of the weaning diet and iron deficiency has been identified in early childhood (Department of Health, 1994). The OPCS infant study reported that less meat (an important source of iron for infants) was given to infants in lower social classes although cost is not given (nor, notably, listed in the questionnaire) as one of the main reasons (White, Freeth and O'Brien, 1992). The MAFF study found that infants who were fed cows' milk or breast milk had significantly lower iron intakes than those whose main milk source was formula milk, with 15% of infants with an iron intake below the Lower Reference Nutrient Intake (LRNI) of 4.2 mg (Mills and Tyler, 1992). Oakley and Rajan found that for a third of mothers (34%), milk was given by adding to tea, with 57% of those in the lowest income group giving their infants tea compared with 15% of those in the highest income group (Oakley and Rajan, 1993). Tea is not advised for infants because tannin binds minerals and can reduce their bio-availability (Department of Health, 1994).

McKillop and Durnin also looked at energy intake and social class differences in a sample of Glasgow infants aged 3 months to 2 years (McKillop and Durnin, 1982). Social class differences were examined using the weighed food intake method in addition to information collected from questionnaires. The highest intake of energy was among female infants in the lowest social class group (unskilled occupations), particularly in the infants under 1 year of age. However, in general, the researchers did not find the kinds of social class variations evident in Oakley and Rajan's study, in either quantity or type of food (McKillop and Durnin, 1982).

Commercial interests

In a referenced review of commercial practices in maternity settings, Mander queries the legality under EC rulings of commercial companies distributing gift packs which include toiletries as well as products relating to bottle feeding (Mander, 1995). Mander notes that the UK laws are less restrictive than in the EU and argues that both the wording in booklets given to mothers in the postpartum period and the promotional activities of commercial companies break EU regulations. The impact on breastfeeding rates and duration of the free distribution of gift packs when mothers are discharged from hospital with their infant has been subject of a series of randomised controlled trials (for example Bergevin, Dougherty and Kramer, 1983; Evans, Lyons and Killien, 1986; Frank *et al.*, 1987; Neifert *et al.*, 1988a), suggesting long-standing concern about the practice.

In an early Canadian trial on this topic, Bergevin and his colleagues (Bergevin, Dougherty and Kramer, 1983) randomised 444 breastfeeding mothers into two groups at discharge group was given a commercial formula sample packet (containing a bottle, formula and related items, including an information booklet) and the other group left the hospital with nothing. Thirty-eight mothers were not interviewed, leaving 406 mothers who were interviewed after 2 months postpartum (the exact length of time after birth is not specified). The study showed no significant differences between those given the formula packet (78% were still breastfeeding at one month postpartum) and those not (84% were still breastfeeding). In sub-analyses of three 'vulnerable groups' (authors' terms), statistical differences were found between the trial group and the controls, with less-educated women, first-time mothers and mothers who had reported illness since leaving hospital being less likely to still be breastfeeding at one month if they had been given a sample. The study also showed that mothers from the overall sample who received the formula packet were more likely than the control mothers to have introduced solids by 2 months postpartum (18% v. 10%), with the differences greater (and in the same direction) in the vulnerable sub-groups (Bergevin, Dougherty and Kramer, 1983).

Three more US randomised controlled trials investigated the same topic. Evans and colleagues randomised their sample of 95 breastfeeding mothers into two groups: those who received formula (dried milk) samples on discharge from hospital, and those who did not. The results from interviews carried out at 6 weeks postpartum showed that there were no statistically significant differences in breastfeeding rates between the two groups (Evans, Lyons and Killien, 1986). Using the same categories of vulnerable groups as Bergevin, Dougherty and Kramer, (1983), Evans and her colleagues studied the effects of the intervention on these groups but unlike Bergevin *et al.* the authors found no statistical differences in duration of breastfeeding (Evans, Lyons and Killien, 1986).

A randomised controlled trial by Neifert *et al.* (1988a) with a sample of 60 first-time adolescent mothers also found no statistically significant differences in breastfeeding duration between a group receiving the 'research gift pack' (which contained no formula) and the control group receiving the commercial gift pack (which contained formula) (Neifert *et al.*, 1988a).

In another US study Frank and colleagues included two interventions in their randomised controlled trial. The first was the introduction of a breastfeeding counsellor and the second, was the replacement of a commercial discharge pack with a non-commercial pack consistent with the WHO code. Various combinations of interventions resulted in three trial groups and a control group (Frank *et al.*, 1987). The authors report that the counselling intervention delayed the introduction of the first solid food to the infant's diet but did not significantly affect the duration of breastfeeding. Those who received the research pack compared to the commercial pack were significantly more likely to prolong exclusive breastfeeding and to feed for longer and to delay the introduction of solids to the infant diet (Frank *et al.*, 1987). Despite the finding from this study, overall the research using randomised controlled trials has not shown a clear effect, in either direction, of the influence of commercial packs on duration of breastfeeding.

The involvement of commercial interests with infant liquid feeding is more clear-cut when the weaning period is under review. Oakley and Rajan, for example, confirm that just under a third of their sample of mothers (29%) had used free samples as a first solid food for their babies (Oakley and Rajan, 1993) and 37% used solid foods as a regular part of their infant's diet in the early months. Mills and Tyler reported that commercial weaning foods were found to be very popular with mothers. Eighty-two per cent of babies had been fed some of these during the survey week of the MAFF study, and such commercial foods contributed more to the diets of the younger infants (aged 6–9 months) than to those of the older infants (9–12 months), for whom 'family foods' gained increasing importance (Mills and Tyler, 1992).

Fuller and Mackie asked women about what they believed to be the origin of the commercial packs they had received in hospital. Ninety-six per cent of the sample of 175 mothers had received such a pack. Fifty-eight per cent recognised that the free samples were from a commercial company. Twenty-two per cent did not know the origin of the pack and nineteen per cent thought that they were from the (hospital) staff (Fuller and Mackie, 1996).

Using commercial foods is not a barrier to good dietary practice, although there may be cost implications which are seldom explored (see Morgan's study in which cost is given as the second most important reason for giving home-prepared foods) (Morgan *et al.*, 1995).

Stordy and colleagues assessed the nutritional values of home prepared baby food; mothers froze a sample of each course prepared for their infants and returned them to the researchers for analysis (Stordy, Redfern and Morgan, 1995), resulting in 265 samples of home prepared weaning food being analysed. The research led the authors to conclude that there was considerable variability of home cooking ranging from poorly to well cooked (i.e. providing more or less nutritional ingredients with vitamins preserved), a variation which is not present in pre-prepared foods (convenience foods) which are more standardised in their nutritional content (Stordy, Redfern and Morgan, 1995).

Knowledge, culture and attitudes

There is an extensive literature on cultural factors affecting infant feeding especially relating to breastfeeding. A highly consistent set of findings, from research carried out over the last fifteen years provides agreement over the central factors in mothers' decision-making. Despite the volume of work in this area, however, studies are not always methodologically strong. A number have used convenience samples, recruiting, for example, from antenatal or prenatal classes. This may lead to over-sampling of 'middle-class' women. Other methodological problems include providing women with a rather emotive list of reasons why they may or may not decide to breastfeed (for example, 'good for baby', 'makes baby healthy') without also providing other options which relate to the woman's social life (for example Neifert *et al.*, 1988b) and studies which ask about breastfeeding intentions without later examining practice (Freed and Fraley, 1993; Maehr *et al.*, 1993).

The most frequently used method is the questionnaire with fixed choice answers. Few researchers have adopted a qualitative approach, and this has led to a series of very repetitive sets of findings, with few studies moving beyond reporting sets of beliefs about breastfeeding. Few researchers, too, are reflective about the potential social pressures which might influence mothers' responses to queries about why they choose not to breastfeed; one exception is McIntosh who remarked that mothers reporting that they had insufficient milk to breastfeed may be a 'socially acceptable response' to support their decision to bottle feed (McIntosh, 1985).

The influence of culture (including social class, region, ethnicity) on breastfeeding is all-important. Morrow and Barraclough (1993) note the considerable variations evident in breastfeeding rates across English-speaking cultures with, for example, 80–95% of Australian mothers breastfeeding on leaving hospital. Thus, in one Australian study, the authors note that '*only* 16% of 10- to 12-month-olds (are) being breastfed' (our emphasis) (Retallack *et al.*, 1994). Similar rates are found in Scandinavia and Poland, while the US, France and Ireland have rates similar to or lower than the UK (Morrow and Barraclough, 1993). A large-scale Canadian study (sample 3120 women) of breastfeeding rates reported that the initial rate of breastfeeding is 69% with the rate at 4 months postpartum being 54.9% (Nolan and Goel, 1995). In the UK, the OPCS national survey demonstrates striking regional, class and age differences in the decision to breastfeed with breastfeeding mothers being of higher social class and older (White, Freeth and O'Brien, 1992). Campbell and Jones report on the range of breastfeeding in Scotland varying between 63% in Orkney, 21% in Lanarkshire and 7.6% in a Glasgow housing estate (Campbell and Jones, 1996).

Although more than fifty per cent of mothers start to breastfeed, the majority cease doing so over the first six months (White, Freeth and O'Brien, 1992). Factors associated with the hospital routines and staff attitudes have been reported above, but the decline in breastfeeding must also be understood in terms of social context and cultural norms. Breastfeeding becomes, for women in some social classes (and neighbourhoods), increasingly a minority behaviour with, at 4 months, 31% and 26% respectively still breastfeeding in social classes IV and V (White, Freeth and O'Brien, 1992) and, in the MAFF study, only 7% breastfeeding after 6 months (Mills and Tyler, 1992).

The social distribution of breastfeeding prevalence has varied during different decades of this century (Wright and Walker, 1983). Recent research has not given us an understanding of class and cultural influences, although the studies of peer experience can be seen as a proxy measure for the more abstract concept of 'culture'. Peer experience is important with a high correlation being reported between the woman's own (or intended) experiences and that of her peers (White, Freeth and O'Brien, 1992; Jones, 1987). McIntosh carried out one of the few interview studies of Scottish women's views on breastfeeding (McIntosh, 1985) and quotes one of his sample from a working-class Scottish culture where bottle feeding predominated: 'It's just that everybody here seems tae dae it (bottle feed) and ah wid feel oot o' place' (McIntosh, 1985, p. 216).

Characteristics of breast feeders

Large-scale national surveys (Mills and Tyler, 1992; White, Freeth and O'Brien, 1992) as well as those with more local samples (Jones, 1987) have indicated a cluster of factors around feeding choice. Thus the most recent OPCS national survey found that having been previously breastfed oneself and having previous experience of breastfeeding are highly correlated with breastfeeding (for example White, Freeth and O'Brien, 1992). Mothers who continued to breastfeed were those in higher social classes, who have previously breastfed a child, were educated beyond the age of 18 and who live in the south of the country.

Those who wish to, and who do maintain breastfeeding are predominantly older women of higher social class, with friends more likely also to breastfeed (White, Freeth and O'Brien, 1992). The social class divisions between types of infant feeding found in this study are marked and are replicated in other work reviewed below.

In a study to ascertain why women abandon breastfeeding at an early stage, Wylie and Verber surveyed women antenatally about their feeding choice and followed them up until 28 days postpartum. This methodological approach allows the researchers to link intention with practice (Wylie and Verber, 1994). They found a strong relationship existed between intention of feeding method with feeding choice at birth, with 68% of those with a firm intention to breastfeed carrying through this method until (at least) 28 days postpartum. They also report that mothers with other children were influenced by their past experiences. Of the 96 mothers who had previously breastfed, 88% successfully breastfeed the present baby (until at least 28 days) while 88% of those who had bottle-fed their previous baby chose to bottle-feed this baby (Wylie and Verber, 1994) (see also Jones, 1987).

US studies have noted similar characteristics of those mothers who breastfeed. In a comparative study of breast and bottle feeders, in a sample of 220 women from Ohio State, the researchers found that breastfeeding women were significantly more likely than bottle feeders to be older, married, with an annual income of over $15 000, to have reached a higher education level, to have planned the pregnancy and to have made an earlier infant feeding decision (Grossman *et al.*, 1990).

These studies are useful in that they strengthen the understanding that the decision about infant feeding is often part of a 'cultural package'. The decision to breastfeed is clearly influenced by social class, age and education (inter-related factors) and previous experience. These factors constitute a strong opportunity for middle-class, older women while those who are younger, with no previous experience of feeding and from working-class (manual) backgrounds, face more barriers. Research into attitudes expands on these opportunities and barriers.

Attitudes to feeding

Few studies offer any details about the mothers' decision-making process in relation to breastfeeding as surveys, in which women are asked to agree to pre-defined statements, constitute the majority of studies in this field. Comparative questionnaire-based surveys of the beliefs of those who breastfed and bottle fed, however, provide some further information about the decision-making of the mothers (for example Manstead, Proffitt and Smart, 1983; Jones, 1987) and provide consistent results. Manstead and colleagues found that mothers who were still breastfeeding six weeks after the birth were significantly more likely to rate the following points about breastfeeding: that it establishes a close bond between mother and baby, that it is good for the mother's figure, that it provides best nourishment for baby and that it protects baby against infection. They were less likely to agree that breastfeeding is embarrassing for the mother and that it limits the mother's social life (Manstead, Proffitt and Smart, 1983). Jones, in a large survey of one district general hospital, using a semi-structured interview schedule, received responses from 1525 women about choice of infant feeding. The most important reason cited in this study by the breast feeders was 'best for baby' (49% of the 681 breast feeders), followed by 'natural' (25%), and 'convenience' (9%) (Jones, 1987).

It is difficult to rank the reasons as to why women chose to breastfeed. Research suggests that mothers may have different reasons. Since each survey uses different wording and takes a slightly different approach, it is not possible to carry out any kind of meta-analysis. Nevertheless, 'best for baby' is cited as an important reason for breastfeeding in a number of studies (for example Jones, 1987; Goodine and Fried, 1984), as is 'protects the baby from disease' (Freed and Fraley, 1993). Findings from other studies suggest that beliefs that breastfeeding is 'natural', 'offers positive satisfaction' are important to women, and that women who have 'positive maternal beliefs' and who are not worried about breastfeeding, are more likely to breastfeed (James, 1981; White, Freeth and O'Brien, 1992; Dusdieker *et al.*, 1985; Woollett, 1987).

While some questionnaires do not necessarily allow women to express doubt or negative views about breastfeeding, Manstead, Proffitt and Smart (1983) and Baisch, Fox and Goldberg (1989) provide two examples of studies where the researchers have included questions which recognised the existence of negative beliefs. Baisch and her colleagues, for example, asked a sample of pregnant adolescents to comment on a series of statements, which included some which were negative. These included 'I have heard from someone who breastfed that breastfeeding hurts' (89% agreement), 'breastfeeding means that I have to eat differently' (54% agreement), and 'breastfeeding makes your breasts sag' (41% agreement) (Baisch, Fox and Goldberg, 1989).

Women who bottle-feed tend to present a different set of priorities. In the study by Manstead and colleagues those women who bottle-fed were statistically more likely than those breastfeeding to agree with the statements relating to the convenience of bottle feeding, that it was a trouble-free feeding method and that it allowed the baby's father to be involved with the feeding (Manstead, Proffitt and Smart, 1983). The view that other people could feed the baby with a bottle (or a variant, the father can feed the baby) was often given as the primary reason in studies using various methods (White, Freeth and O'Brien, 1992; McIntosh, 1985; Gabriel, Gabriel and Lawrence, 1986). Jones's large sample included 844 bottle feeders, who gave priority to convenience (26%), with not liking the idea of breastfeeding (18%), and embarrassment (13%) as other responses; less than one per cent mentioned sharing feeding with husband (Jones, 1987). The findings from these studies suggest that women have different priorities when deciding upon infant feeding; the breast feeders reported the well-known benefits (for example, good for baby) while in general the bottle-feeders were more concerned about others being able to feed, and held negative feelings about breastfeeding. These potential opportunities and barriers are elaborated in further research.

The literature also contains reports from women that breastfeeding is not always straightforward and that there may be perceived or actual problems with its accomplishment. Reasons for giving up were often focused specifically upon the mechanics of feeding, including (perceived) insufficient milk, not knowing how much the baby was getting, engorgement and sore nipples as well as other factors such as illness of mother or baby (Beeken and Waterston, 1992; White, Freeth and O'Brien, 1992; McIntosh, 1985; James, 1981; Lilburne *et al.*, 1988; Salt *et al.*, 1994).

Breastfeeding is a biologically 'natural' activity; the World Health Organisation (WHO) suggest that only 1–5% of women in industrialised countries are physiologically incapable of sustaining breastfeeding (WHO, 1989). Nevertheless studies reported in this review have suggested that some mothers may experience practical problems in establishing the process, while Morrow and Barraclough (among others) have also noted that real or perceived problems are frequently recorded (Morrow and Barraclough, 1993). The extent to which women experience such difficulties, the level and reasons for their commitment to this practice and the kind of support they feel that they receive should be considered in more detail. Sensitivity to this issue by health professionals would be important, since this must constitute a very definite barrier.

An Australian study, where the rate of breastfeeding is somewhat higher than in the UK, focused only upon bottle-feeders (Lilburne *et al.*, 1988). This study reported, too, that 'insufficient milk' was the main reason for the mothers to switch to bottle feeding. The authors also questioned mothers about how they constituted the bottle feeds and from this evidence (alone) noted that a proportion of mothers appeared to be making errors in mixing the feed, with about a sixth of the mothers making up a formula which was too concentrated (Lilburne *et al.*, 1988).

Breastfeeding and embarrassment

Surveys and interviews studies have confirmed the view that some women are not happy with the idea of breastfeeding. Not liking the idea of breastfeeding and embarrassment are important barriers to women adopting breastfeeding on a longer-term basis, the latter offered by only 7% of mothers in the OPCS survey, but found to be a major factor in other research (for example James, 1981; Manstead, Proffitt and Smart, 1983; Wright and Walker, 1983; McIntosh, 1985; Jones, 1987). McIntosh's study of first-time Scottish mothers, already noted above, is one of the few which have used qualitative methods (McIntosh, 1985). The sample of 69 working-class mothers was interviewed on six occasions beginning during pregnancy and ending after the infant was 9 months of age. Respondents reported that social unacceptableness and inconvenience of breastfeeding were the prime reasons for bottle feeding (McIntosh, 1985). The lack of acceptability was bound up with notions that breasts were essentially sexual objects and that using them to feed the infant was 'distasteful' (McIntosh, 1985) (see also Gregg's study of school pupils described below) (Gregg, 1989).

Privacy

Several studies have investigated the issue of privacy when breastfeeding (Hally *et al.*, 1984; McIntosh, 1985; Gregg, 1989). Living in the parental home was a barrier to breastfeeding, particularly to single women for whom embarrassment was a more important factor than for married women (McIntosh, 1985; Hally *et al.*, 1984). McIntosh notes that the concern with privacy was underlined by the finding that those of his sample who were living in their own homes were more likely to breastfeed, while those living with parents or other relatives were less likely to make this decision (McIntosh, 1985).

In Gregg's survey of fourth-year pupils attending a UK comprehensive school, the adolescents' views about privacy were striking (Gregg, 1989). Gregg found that only a relatively small proportion of the sample (18%) had been breastfed (36% did not know). Forty per cent of the girls and 28% of boys had seen a relative breastfeeding. While 100% of both genders thought that their own infant could be breastfed at home, percentages dropped in response to the idea of breastfeeding with the baby's father present (87% boys, 81% girls) or with female family members present (approximately 50%) (Gregg, 1989).

A Canadian study by Ellis asked very similar questions of a sample of school pupils (girls and boys) from 8th–12th grade (adolescents), although the sampling strategy in this study was somewhat weaker than that of Gregg, drawing from nine schools and across a range of grades to recruit 408 students (Ellis, 1983). From the responses the author reports that 72% had seen a relative or friend breastfeeding and 43% said that they themselves were breastfed, a rather higher percentage than in the UK study. Ninety per cent of girls and boys thought that breastfeeding at home was 'acceptable' for one's future infant, but only 68.7% thought this was acceptable 'in presence of family' (Ellis, 1983).

Breastfeeding in public

If breastfeeding in front of relatives is perceived to be embarrassing, breastfeeding in public places was even less acceptable, although in one study, those who had previously witnessed breastfeeding were less likely to be opposed to it (System Three for HEBS, 1994). The school pupils from Gregg's and Ellis's respective studies felt that breastfeeding in public was not very acceptable with, in Gregg's Liverpool study, less than 5% reporting that they saw it as acceptable to breastfeed in the park, shopping mall or on the bus (Gregg, 1989) and in Ellis' study less than a quarter responding positively to breastfeeding in these public places (Ellis, 1983).

In a news section of the journal the *Health Visitor* reference is made to the British Tourist Authority's leaflet 'Days Out in 1996' which includes the following text: 'Please note that breastfeeding in public is not considered generally acceptable' (*Health Visitor*, September 1996). However, in the NOP survey for the Royal College of Midwives it was found that 75% of high street restaurants surveyed provided satisfactory, good or very good facilities for breastfeeding (cited in Laurent, 1993). Attitudes such as those expressed above should be seen as important barriers, even to those who successfully breastfeed. There are, as noted, important social class and other factors related to those who choose to, and those who choose not to breastfeed. However, the negative views about breastfeeding in public places may be viewed as a barrier raised not only by cultural subgroups but more generally by wider social attitudes.

Partners' views on feeding method

The partner or husband's views on feeding choice, and the role of social support in the decision to breastfeed are important aspects which influence successful breastfeeding (Matich and Sims, 1992; Jones, 1987; Freed and Fraley, 1993; Wylie and Verber, 1994). The National Opinion Poll (NOP) carried out a survey for the Royal College of Midwives (cited by Laurent, 1993) and ascertained the views of 924 men on the topic of breastfeeding in public. Laurent reports that half of the men objected to women breastfeeding their infant in 'any place they chose', while 14% of the sample found the idea of breastfeeding in public unacceptable (Laurent, 1993). Voss's pilot study sample of male partners reported a similar percentage. In the same study, nearly half the men said that although they were consulted about infant feeding, their partner had made the final decision (Voss, Finnis and Manners, 1993).

Freed and Fraley focused specifically upon the relationship between the father's attitude and the mother's feeding plans, surveying the mothers prenatally (Freed and Fraley, 1993). The study findings are that 70% of mothers planned to breastfeed and (as other studies have also shown, for example Matich and Sims, 1992) these mothers were more knowledgeable about feeding choice and were more likely to predict positive attitudes of the fathers towards breastfeeding (Freed and Fraley, 1993). Such findings are difficult to interpret in this study since the study population was biased towards middle-class mothers who are statistically more likely to choose breastfeeding and, since the study was carried out antenatally, is only *predictive* of the fathers' attitudes. Nevertheless, other studies confirm that breastfeeding women were more likely to have gained support about their feeding choice from the baby's father or their friends during pregnancy than were bottle-feeders (Grossman *et al.*, 1990) and that active support from professionals and friends has been shown to be important (see Salt *et al.*, 1994; Wylie and Verber, 1994).

Although there is a wealth of surveys on attitudes towards infant feeding, and considerable consistency in the findings, one may conclude that much about the social processes and decision-making within this area remains opaque. Thus it is impossible to know the manner in which the (middle-class) partner, or the media, for example, may influence feeding choice. Given the strong social class pressures, it would be important to understand the difficulties faced by some women from backgrounds where breastfeeding is not common. There is also a dearth of studies which have reported, in more detail, on the satisfactions and the constraints with either form of liquid feeding, the opportunities presented by each method and the impact of part-time or full-time work on feeding.

Weaning

Although the area of women's decisions regarding liquid feeding has attracted considerable attention, there are fewer studies of attitudes and beliefs about weaning. Two large-scale national studies have reported on weaning and the weaned infant (White, Freeth and O'Brien, 1992; Mills and Tyler, 1992), while there is a small group of studies which deal in part with infants' food intake and in part with social factors which correlate with particular diets (Persson and Samuelson, 1985; McIntosh, 1986; Oakley and Rajan, 1993; Morgan *et al.*, 1995). The McIntosh study stands alone as the only qualitative study on the topic. One further study by Retallack *et al.* (1994) on infant feeding practices is included in this discussion as the findings relate to the general topic.

Although Department of Health recommendations suggest weaning should not take place before 4 months, and that all babies should receive a mixed diet by 6 months (Department of Health, 1994), the literature reports wide variation in weaning with the majority of infants being weaned earlier than recommended. The MAFF-funded study reported that the average age at which babies are weaned is 13 weeks with a range of 3–32 weeks (Mills and Tyler, 1992). Nineteen per cent of babies in the OPCS study were weaned at 8 weeks (White, Freeth and O'Brien,

1992). In McIntosh's study, 56% of infants were weaned by 8 weeks (McIntosh, 1986). The link between bottle feeding and earlier weaning has been noted frequently, suggesting a cluster of attitudes around the issue of infant feeding. Few studies have examined in any detail why mothers chose to wean early although McIntosh's study with Scottish working-class women (reported above) suggests that women held positive cultural attitudes about plumpness in a baby as an indication of wellbeing and of mother's love (McIntosh, 1986).

What emerges from more detailed studies of solid infant feeding (although often on *reported* intake rather than actual diet) is a mixture of good intentions on the part of the mother, and practices which contravene the most recent Department of Health recommendations on the infant diet. In a large-scale quantitative study with a quota sample of 1004 mothers with infants between 3 and 12 months, Morgan and her colleagues studied mothers' attitudes towards 'healthy eating' for infants (Morgan *et al.*, 1995). Many mothers reported thinking about their child's nutrient intake and adapting an adult diet to avoid giving their infant particular foods. Aspects of the infant's diet which mothers considered to be very important included giving infants a variety of foods and plenty to drink and achieving a low sugar and salt intake. One-fifth of mothers felt that giving the infant plenty of calories was not an important consideration, while 83% of mothers felt that a high fibre intake and 87% a low fat intake were either very important or important (Morgan *et al.*, 1995). Over 80% of the sample were fed home-prepared foods although most parents used both these and manufactured foods. When asked about reasons for giving home-prepared baby foods, 65% agreed with the proposition that they believed them to be nutritionally superior to manufactured foods, 48% agreed that cost was important and 31% gave convenience as a reason (Morgan and Stordy, 1995).

Although not an attitudinal study, one Australian study (Retallack *et al.*, 1994) reported similar practices, although their sampling strategy was weaker, relying upon volunteers in Adelaide shopping complexes who were asked about their weaning practices with their infant (infants aged up to and including 52 weeks old). The authors noted that the majority of practices were compatible with South Australian guidelines but the study findings are quite similar to UK studies with 40% of infants being weaned under the age of 4 months (Retallack *et al.*, 1994). The authors expressed concern about the infants' iron intake, with the mothers reportedly increasingly offering cows' milk after the infant was 6 months old. In several UK studies a small proportion of mothers reported giving their infant semi-skimmed milk and a tiny number skimmed milk (Mills and Tyler, 1992; White, Freeth and O'Brien, 1992), practices which are appropriate for an adult diet but not in line with government recommendations on the infant diet (Department of Health, 1994).

Several studies reported that, even before the infants were 1 year old, they were already being given a range of foods. For example, in the MAFF study, yoghurts, biscuits, sweets, chocolate and potato crisps were reported popular with the older sample (9–12 months) (Mills and Tyler, 1992). Oakley and Rajan, in the detailed questionnaire survey reviewed above, documented the 'junk food' content (authors' term) of the infant's diet as reported by the mothers. Sixty-three per cent of babies were given at least one portion of sweets, biscuits, cakes, crisps, ice-cream, orange squash or fizzy drinks in the course of a day (Oakley and Rajan, 1993). The researchers provided evidence that the proportion of 'healthy foods' (authors' term) eaten by the infants increased with income and education, in owner-occupier households and among those with a larger number of household amenities (Oakley and Rajan, 1993).

Retallack and colleagues reported in the Australian study that a minority of infants were being given non-fortified adult cereals, and foods high in sugar and salt (Retallack *et al.*, 1994). These findings were reflected in the MAFF study where, of those infants who ate potatoes only, 39% of mothers added salt and of those who ate vegetables (but not potatoes) 36% added salt to them. One-third of infants consumed breakfast cereals with sugar added in the home and 45% of mothers who gave their infants milk-based dishes sweetened them with sugar (Mills and Tyler, 1992).

Baby fruit juices are widely used as infant drinks (Mills and Tyler, 1992; Oakley and Rajan, 1993) and their suitability depends on how often they are given and the amount of sugar that they contain. Mothers are more likely to give their 6-week-old babies unsweetened drinks in 1990 compared to 1985, but the proportion of mothers giving sweetened herbal drinks has increased since 1985. By about 9 months of age, water, unsweetened baby drinks and herbal drinks were the most popular drinks, but 22% of babies were receiving baby drinks with sugar or glucose (White, Freeth and O'Brien, 1992). The study by Persson and colleagues stands out as one of the few which looked at infant diet and dental caries, arguing that the link between sugar in the diet and future dental caries was already established through a dietary pattern at the age of 1, when the Swedish children were first studied (Persson *et al.*, 1985).

In Morgan and her colleagues' study, 29% of mothers reported that they gave their infant vitamin supplements, although since the majority of infants were under 6 months old they therefore did not need supplementation (Morgan and Stordy, 1995). In the MAFF study 45% of infants were given dietary supplements, 43% of these being in the form of vitamin drops; almost a quarter of mothers received these under the Welfare Food Scheme, the remaining proportion purchasing them at the clinic (Mills and Tyler, 1992). Vitamin supplements were not mentioned by Oakley and Rajan (1993) or McIntosh (1986).

These studies do not report extensively on attitudes and culture, but rather emphasise that, despite good intentions, a significant proportion of infants are being fed foods which are not necessarily appropriate for their age group.

Sources of professional advice

Four UK studies included questions about sources of advice as a part of a larger project (Oakley and Rajan, 1993; McIntosh, 1986; Morgan and Stordy, 1995; Fuller and Mackie, 1996) and two small studies have examined the topic in its own right (Chalmers, 1991; Walker, 1995). Oakley and Rajan found that on feeding issues the majority of mothers (73%) used their own experience although 58% also reported the health visitor as a source of advice (mothers could list more than one source) (Oakley and Rajan, 1993). In an analysis which took 'housing tenure' as the index of social class, the researchers reported that a high proportion of middle-class mothers, and those women with only one other child, named the health visitor as a source of advice. They also cited books and magazines as a major source of advice (Oakley and Rajan, 1993).

McIntosh's findings confirm this study. In the study referenced earlier, about one-fifth of the women reported a preference for professional advice and adhered to formal recommendations about weaning (McIntosh, 1986). However McIntosh reported that, among his working-class sample, professional advice conflicted with lay sources and that, for over three-quarters of the sample (79%), practical experience was seen as more relevant than the 'textbook knowledge' of professionals, a trend which was not helped by health visitors reportedly giving advice without explanation. The liking for lay rather than professional advice was seen to be part of a more general preference for informal advice in relation to infant care (McIntosh, 1986).

However, other studies (all questionnaire-based) report that the health visitor emerged as the most cited source. Morgan and Stordy found that 60% of their sample said that the health visitor was the most influential person after the infant's birth in relation to advice about solid foods. Thirty-six per cent cited experience with previous infants and 18% information from books and magazines (Morgan and Stordy, 1995).

Fuller and Mackie (1996) found that the health visitor was the source of advice followed by the largest proportion of their sample. Thirty-nine per cent followed their health visitors' advice, with 14% following advice from a family member, and 13% using books or magazines. Health visitors were regarded by a substantial minority of the sample as unbiased sources of information. Thirty-nine per cent of mothers thought that samples of commercially produced foods given by the clinic were more likely to be 'healthy' (authors' term) than others received through the post or in magazines (Fuller and Mackie, 1996).

Walker took a convenience sample of 76 first-time mothers whose infants were between the age of 6 and 9 months at the time of study (Walker, 1995). The results of her study confirm the finding of the majority of other studies reported above, that the health visitor was the source of advice most frequently mentioned (83% of the sample), followed by mother (75%), friends (74%), and books and magazines (72%). Walker notes from open-ended comments that mothers were aware that their practice was not always in line with professional and official recommendations ('I do not think he would have been so happy and content if I had taken the health visitor's advice not to give solids until 12 weeks'; 'Official recommendations are only guidelines. Too many dos and don'ts instead of using common sense') (Walker, 1995, p. 110).

Chalmers' telephone survey was set up to examine the consistency of advice given to breastfeeding mothers discharged into the community by community midwives and health visitors (Chalmers, 1991). The study is too slight to place much weight on the findings (very small sample, 9 community midwives and 31 health visitors, with very short telephone interviews) but even within these limitations clear differences between the two groups emerged. The community midwives reported more intra-group consistency in their advice (Chalmers, 1991). This study is unusual in that it recognises that intra-professional variation may cause problems and anxieties for women. Larger-scale studies would help us understand the nature of the variation and ways in which it could be reduced.

This is not a strong area of research, with relatively few studies on attitudes and beliefs, and rather more on feeding practices. What is suggested by this research (and there is really not sufficient evidence to say more) is that mothers appear to be thoughtful about the diet of their infant. This could form a positive basis for further education. The research suggests that mothers do not necessarily understand the underlying nutritional messages regarding an infant's diet and that professional help is not always seen as appropriate because such advice is not always in keeping with lay attitudes and beliefs. It may be that more effective forms of professional intervention should be explored bearing in mind, in particular, the cultural barriers towards seeking and acting upon professional advice by some women. These are important areas for attention when considering future interventions in dietary change.

Babies do not only receive food in the home, as increasing numbers of babies attend day-care facilities such as workplace crèches, nurseries and childminders. Earlier dietary guidelines paid little attention to the under-5s and in response to this the London Food Commission produced guidelines in 1985 for staff in charge of under-5s' facilities. The Department of Health produced a report on infant feeding in 1988 which contained guidelines on diets for the under-5s although not in a practical form appropriate for staff at day-care facilities. The most recent report produced by the Department of Health recommends that consistent written or video educational materials on weaning should be used to communicate information to nurseries, playgroups and the public at large (Department of Health, 1994).

4. Children aged 1–5 years

Introduction

This section is concerned with research on children aged between 1 and 5 years. Research does not follow the themes of the previous section on infant feeding (for example, by examining details of the young children's diet and attitudes towards the foods) but starts with a fresh agenda, providing little opportunity to link back to research findings from the field of infant feeding. Few studies provide detailed information about children's dietary intake, and much of our knowledge of the eating habits of young children rests with the study described in Appendix B by Gregory *et al.* (1995). Much of the work described within this section is concerned with ways in which children's food preferences are formed. Research in the area of young children and eating behaviours derives largely from psychology, with experimental methods dominating the work. Very few studies reported below have examined the social and cultural context of children's eating through qualitative work and with interviews with mothers; however, the social context of decisions about food choice is recognised by the work carried out on television advertisements.

In this field, many studies derive their information about young children from the parents (often the mother) rather than the young child. These data are seen in the social sciences as acceptable proxy data, children of this age often being thought to be too young to be personally involved with surveys and interviews. There are exceptions, however, such as the Canadian studies of 'breakfast skipping' which are geared to the involvement of young children (McIntyre, 1993; McIntyre and Horbul, 1995) and the large number of experimental studies carried out on children approximately aged between 2 and 5 years (for example, see the work of Birch and her colleagues) (Birch *et al.*, 1987; 1991).

Research which focuses upon *family* eating patterns does necessarily separate out, as in this report, women's nutritional patterns and those of their children; thus some of the studies reviewed in the section on 'women of childbearing age' cover issues concerning mothers *and* their young children (for example Charles and Kerr, 1986; Mayall, 1986; Dowler and Calvert, 1995). Relevant findings from these studies are reported below.

There are other clusters of studies in this sub-section which use a variety of methods, including content analysis of television (Warnke and Albrecht, 1994), videotaping of family life (Koivisto, Fellenius and Sjøden, 1994) and experimental studies (Birch *et al.*, 1987). This latter genre of studies, of experimental format and usually carried out in a laboratory or study room, provide ways of manipulating the child's environment in order to ascertain the key factors which guide the child's food choices (for example, taste preferences, time of day). These studies are important because they focus upon young children's eating preferences and thus are highly relevant to this review. This category of research derives predominantly from the US, although, with volunteer subjects and with small samples (usually below 30 individuals). The complicated design and small number of subjects (often volunteers) place certain question marks about the validity of the conclusions. UK researchers have criticised their lack of social context and argued that this and the US bias raises concerns about the generalisability of the findings to the UK (Young and Hetherington, 1996).

Access

A major barrier to healthy eating has been reported to be limited income (for example Dowler and Calvert, 1995). The restricted diet reported for women living in poverty is equally true for young children. Thus, for example, Taylor and Koblinski showed, in their survey of 73 homeless mothers, that their pre-school children (aged between 3 and 5 years) consumed a diet high in sugar (Taylor and Koblinski, 1994). The same US children ate a diet which was deficient in the number of servings of dairy products, fruit and vegetables and grain products. The only adequate aspect of their diet was that of meat and meat products (Taylor and Koblinski, 1994). Drake (1992) studied a sample of 96 homeless single women and their children (age range 1–10 years), living in two shelters using weighed food records, anthropometric measures, biochemical indices and interviews; Drake reports that the diets were high in fats and low in iron, with intake about 50% of the (US) RDA for all age groups (Drake, 1992).

UK research provides further evidence that the diets of children may be restricted when resources are scarce; thus in the NCH study reviewed earlier in the report one in ten children under the age of 5 had gone without food during the last month because of lack of money (NCH, 1991); however, other factors also affect the child's nutritional intake and nearly one in four children in this study had gone without food during the last month because they did not like the food on offer (NCH, 1991). Risk minimisation strategies are particularly important in these circumstances. For example, one strategy illustrated by Dobson and colleagues (and others) is for mothers not to experiment with food which the children do not like, or where their preferences are unknown, as in either case this could lead to wastage (Dobson *et al.*, 1994). Thus children's preferences, even with very young children, are perceived as being of considerable importance when food is being purchased. This is discussed at greater length below.

The benefits for mothers with children of having private transport were underlined by Mayall, who provided evidence from her interview study that the advantages go beyond simply being able to have access to a wider choice of food outlets (Mayall, 1986). Middle-class women in Mayall's sample commented that a car made shopping easier and quicker, and that this ease of access gave mothers more time to spend with their children. Women also reported that child control was easier for these reasons, and mothers did not have to give their children food to keep them quiet. Mayall contrasts this with accounts from working-class mothers who found that the difficulties of access to shops led them to 'bribe' the child with sweets (for example, waiting in a bus queue with a bored child) (Mayall, 1986). Mayall's study brings out very clearly the way in which 'access' factors can create opportunities for, or barriers to, families with different resources; transport is a key issue and one which has been neglected in previous studies of the social context of food consumption. This area does require more research in order to explore the experiences of mothers from different social backgrounds in more detail.

Television and advertising – what effect on children's food choice?

Recognition that the media are influential in food choice has led to a cohort of studies which have analysed the content of Saturday morning television food advertising which is aimed at young children (for example Warnke and Albrecht, 1994; Kotz and Story, 1994). These studies are included as the media are recognised as important in shaping attitudes towards foods.

Warnke and Albrecht carried out a content analysis of children's television, recording every third Saturday throughout three months on three major networks (Warnke and Albrecht, 1994) (as well as looking at food advertising in magazines). Their analysis showed that the vast majority of television food advertisements (97.1%) fell into the 'food use' category. When these foods were divided into food groups, fruit was mentioned 27% of the time and vegetables only 3.7% of the time on television. Breads and cereals were mentioned 29.5% of the time and pre-sweetened cereals accounted for 70% of the cereals mentioned or shown from this group. Potatoes, including French fries and 'tater tots' were the vegetable most often mentioned or shown; the fruits most often mentioned or shown were apples, bananas, pears, oranges/orange juice, strawberries and grapes which were usually included as part of a complete/balanced breakfast or as flavours (Warnke and Albrecht, 1994).

Using similar techniques in another US study, Kotz and Story recorded Saturday morning television commercials on five networks for three Saturdays, resulting in 52½ hours of television advertisements (Kotz and Story, 1994). Of the 997 commercials that were shown 56.5% were for food. Just under half (43.6%) of these were for foods classified in the 'fats, oils and sweets' food group, and the next largest proportion (37.5%) was categorised into the 'bread, cereals, rice and pasta' group, of which 23% were high sugar cereals (Kotz and Story, 1994). From their analysis Kotz and Story report that advertisements for fruits and vegetables were virtually non-existent. The authors concluded that the majority of commercials shown during Saturday mornings promoted foods which were predominantly high in fats and/or sugar, many of which had a relatively low nutritional value and that 'the diet presented on Saturday morning television is the antithesis of what is recommended as healthy eating for children' (Kotz and Story, 1994).

Using a sample of 66 mothers with at least one child aged between 3 and 8 years, Taras and his colleagues questioned the mothers about the food requests and television viewing preferences of one of their children (Taras *et al.*, 1989). Sugared cereals stood out as the food item most requested by the children and most often purchased. Overall, the study showed a strong relationship between food groups (categorised for the study into high fat/sugar/salt, low fat/sugar/salt) which mothers reported the child requesting and the food groups shown on the television advertisements. This US study used a population which was two-thirds Hispanic and methods which could incorporate a number of biases (in recall, for example), but suggests as other studies have, that there is some relationship between television advertising of certain foods and children's preferences (Taras *et al.*, 1989).

Taras and his colleagues carried out a further study following new US regulations in 1990, which limited the amount of commercial time allowed on children's television (Taras and Gage, 1995). The researchers videotaped and analysed a full week of television shown at children's viewing times on seven channels. Commercial advertising accounted for 16% of children's total viewing time, with 47.8% relating to food (products, beverages and restaurants). Of advertised cereals, the large proportion of advertisements was for cereals high in sugar (84.6%). One hundred per cent of sweets' advertisements were high in sugar and 40.1% were high in fat; the majority of beverages were sweetened (83.2%). The authors conclude that although the proportion of time spent on food commercials has decreased over twenty years, commercials for foods of poor nutritional value still account for a large proportion of children's televised viewing (Taras and Gage, 1995).

However, other studies using a more experimental technique have seldom been able to show a close relationship between the television commercials and the consumption of particular foods. Jeffrey and his colleagues set up a series of experiments to ascertain whether there was a link between television commercials watched and subsequent increased consumption of foods (Jeffrey, McLellarn and Fox, 1982). The researchers involved 47 4- and 5-year-olds randomly assigning them to three groups, 'low-nutrition', 'pro-nutrition' and 'non-food control'. The children were first administered the behavioural eating test (the BET test which involved food choice and food consumption) and a food attitude scale. A week later the researchers showed the different groups 'low-nutritional' and 'pro-nutritional' (their terms) advertisements and applied the tests again to the children. They subsequently analysed the findings to see if there were pre- and post-test variations on the children's scores. The study did not provide strong conclusions although the authors noted that low nutritional advertising increased recall and consumption of low nutrition foods (i.e. the post-test scores for consumption showed a significant increase). The authors noted that the pro-nutritional advertisements had less impact in the study, but were in real life typically produced with small budgets compared with the large budgets of the low-nutrition advertisements. Furthermore, because more of the television advertisements were low-nutrition type the children had less exposure to high-nutritional advertising both in the experimental situation and during their normal television viewing (Jeffrey, McLellarn and Fox, 1982). In a further experiment using the same methods, but with groups of 4- and 9-year-olds, the researchers found that age did not affect consumption but that gender did, with more of the boys consuming low-nutritional foods than the girls (Jeffrey, McLellarn and Fox, 1982).

Also using the BET, Peterson and her colleagues have shown that young children (in this study the sample of children had an average age of 6.2 years but included 5-year-olds) learned 'pro-nutritional' (the researchers' term) constructs as they were presented on videotapes (Peterson *et al.*, 1984). The study showed that children's scores increased significantly on 'recall' and 'information' measures but showed no change on 'preference' or 'consumption', the study suggesting that children may remember messages but do not always act on them.

Gorn and Goldberg's study focused upon the effect of daily exposure of children to certain items on television, taking a sample of 72 children (aged between 5 and 8 years) at a summer camp and, therefore, whose access to television was controlled (Gorn and Goldberg, 1982). In this study, four groups of children were shown four different 'messages' (sweets commercials, commercial messages, fruit commercials and public service announcements) during cartoon programmes, after which they were led to another part of the room where snack choices were available to them. The snacks fell into different types of foods (fruit and sweets) and drinks (fruit juice and sweetened drinks). Gorn and Goldberg report that those who viewed the sweets advertisements were more likely to pick sweets as snacks and less likely to pick fruit, while those exposed to fruit juice advertisements were most likely to pick fruit juice (Gorn and Goldberg, 1982). The authors comment, as have others, on the familiarity of children with sweets advertisements.

The lack of clear trends and the strong US bias in the research makes it difficult to generalise from the findings. The various researchers, too, have noted the difficulty of studying the impact of television advertising in this experimental manner, since even with young children the familiarity of television may influence the experimental conditions. In a review of the literature on advertising and children's food choice, however, Young and Hetherington argue for caution in this area of research (Young and Hetherington, 1996), and question studies which imply causality between television advertisements and children's food requests. The authors confirmed the methodological soundness of Galst and White's early study which showed that, if a child is interested and enjoyed commercials, this resulted in more supermarket requests (Galst and White, 1976). However, it could also be suggested that there is evidence that children's food choices can be influenced by changing the food messages shown on television and that the *potential* for change should make children's television an important forum for future interventions.

Knowledge, culture, attitudes

A 'proper meal'

Many families now report that they sit down to eat together only a limited number of times each week (Murcott, 1997). Other studies have highlighted adolescent 'grazing' habits (Anderson, Macintyre and West, 1993). Research has suggested that changing eating patterns are affected not only by who prepares the food but also what kind of meal it is and with whom the family members eat. The limited research on the interplay between these factors allows us to begin to appreciate the implications for women and children's 'healthy eating'.

There is considerable discussion which concerns the status and nature of 'a proper meal' (Murcott, 1983; Mayall, 1986; Charles and Kerr, 1988). In separate studies, using interviews with women about their family's eating habits, Murcott (1983) and Mayall (1986) have reported that a 'proper meal' involves the family sitting down together to eat, and serves a range of social functions including that of socialising children into how to behave when eating and that of allowing social intercourse to take place (Murcott, 1997). From the research, the definition of a 'proper meal' is that it consists of meat, (sometimes fish), potatoes and vegetables (Charles and Kerr, 1988), a definition which would adequately meet the recommendations laid out in Department of Health recommendations (Department of Health, 1991). In Charles and Kerr's interview study mothers reported that a 'proper meal' was produced as the main meal of the day, and that other meals did not follow the same 'rules' (Charles and Kerr, 1988). Charles and Kerr also note that it was seen as important by their respondents that a *woman* cooks the meal for it to be seen as a 'proper meal' (Charles and Kerr, 1988). Of interest is the finding that 47% of their sample reported that they ate differently when one adult member of the family was absent from the meal and were far more likely to produce snacks or convenience foods, usually as requested by the children (Charles and Kerr, 1988). This finding is also reported by Mayall (1986).

These findings, drawn from only a handful of studies, suggest complexity with the components of a meal based not only upon the category (snack, main meal) but also who prepared it and who was present. Nutritionally, the research suggests that there is a cultural acceptance of particular food combinations, and that the desire by many mothers to produce a 'proper meal' on some days a week is an opportunity for them and the children to eat a balanced meal. Nevertheless, the literature which is concerned with young children and family eating habits suggests that family members may have varying food preferences and that the 'outcome' of the meal, that is what is eaten during a particular time period defined as meal-time, is the result of complex social processes which are discussed below.

A series of studies on breakfast eating is relevant under this heading. Breakfast is a meal which has been identified as nutritionally important in the literature (Hill, 1995). In the 1962 Iowa Breakfast Series, the morning meal was defined as a meal which provided a quarter of the daily calories and the daily protein needs and ready-to-eat breakfast cereals were identified as the best source of daily iron and B vitamins. Culturally it has significance in this section of the review as it is suggested that breakfast is the first meal in which young children may cater for themselves (Hill, 1995).

Two studies from different Canadian states (McIntyre, 1993; McIntyre and Horbul, 1995) report on breakfast eating and type of foods consumed at breakfast with a large, cross-sectional survey of young schoolchildren (1st–3rd grade). The studies were carried out in two states with a sample of over 2000 children attending primary schools in Nova Scotia (the survey was carried out twice within a month with slightly different sample sizes each time) (McIntyre, 1993) and 4079 in North-eastern Ontario (McIntyre and Horbul, 1995). In both instances the survey (using the Halifax Breakfast Survey Instrument, which is largely pictorial) was administered by a videotaped puppet which took the children through the instructions and provided the opportunity for non-participation. In Nova Scotia, the median breakfast skipping rate was 4.8%, that is children coming to school without eating or drinking anything on the study morning. Breakfast skipping was significantly higher in children from grade 1 than grade 3 and boys were more likely to skip breakfast than girls; younger children were less likely to have what the researcher defined as a 'vigorously adequate' breakfast than the older children (McIntyre, 1993). One-third of children prepared their own breakfasts and these were significantly more likely to be boys, to be in a higher grade and to eat more cereal, chips, fizzy drinks and coffee than children who had someone else to prepare their foods (McIntyre, 1993). In the second study in schools in Ontario (McIntyre and Horbul, 1995) similar methods produced similar results in relation to age and proportion of breakfast skippers.

Cornelius studied breakfast eating as part of a broader examination of health habits of school-age children (aged 5–17 years) in a large-scale survey of disadvantaged children ($n = 6722$) (Cornelius, 1991). The study, using reports from parents, contradicted the gender differences identified by McIntyre, with girls less likely to eat breakfast than boys, and a significant variation in breakfast eating by education of head of household, with 83.6% of children in college-educated families eating breakfast regularly compared to 72.9% of those where the head of household was not a high school graduate (Cornelius, 1991).

What is increasingly obvious from the literature, too, is that families do not necessarily eat their meals sitting round a table. Eating in front of the television (Charles and Kerr, 1988) and snacking (Mayall, 1986) are just two forms of food consumption which are reported. It is not only adolescents who 'snack'. Children snack from an early age (see Seagren and Terry, 1991 below). Mothers, in the study carried out by Dobson *et al.*, reported that their children were teased at school if they did not have the same snacks (such as crisps and chocolate) as others did (Dobson *et al.*, 1994). Dobson and her colleagues report that the pressures to purchase such food was considerable for mothers with low incomes.

Children's tastes

There is evidence (Gregory *et al.*, 1995) to suggest that young children do not always eat food of high nutritional quality. The understanding that children's taste preferences are established when they are very young dominates much research with small children. The pioneering work of Clara Davis in the 1920s and 1930s led to the interpretation that, given a wide variety of choice, children had a 'natural' ability to create a diet which was balanced in food stuffs (Davis, 1928). Researchers have argued subsequently that the young children in these classic studies were exposed only to fresh, unprocessed foods and not to the range of foods now common in the Western world and that the results should be viewed with caution (Story and Brown, 1987). More recently Birch and her co-workers (Birch *et al.*, 1991) carried out a similar experiments with 15 children aged between 2 and 5 years on six days, in a study designed to investigate meal-to-meal and day-to-day variations in the food intake in young children. The researchers concluded, as had Davis, that 'the successful feeding of children is best accomplished by providing them with a variety of healthful foods and allowing them to eat what they wished' (Birch *et al.*, 1991, p. 235). Nevertheless, these authors recognise the complexities surrounding the food intake of young children.

In a study with a poorly constructed sample but a strong effect (Klesges *et al.*, 1991) children were asked to decide upon what to eat from a table with foods from different food groups (classified by the researchers as 'low', 'medium' and 'high' in nutritional value). From the volunteer sample of 53 children (mean age 5.9 years), children were allowed to choose the foods they wanted to eat for their lunch and to place the foods on a tray. The foods were then returned to the table and the children told to repeat the task but that their mother was about to come into the room. The experiment revealed that telling the children that parental involvement was imminent decreased considerably the sugar content of foods selected (Klesges *et al.*, 1991).

Experimental studies (for example Birch and Marlin, 1982; Pelchat and Pliner, 1995) have attempted, under laboratory conditions, to isolate why children choose certain foods. Thus Birch and her colleagues (Birch and Marlin, 1982) in two experiments with 2-year-old children, offered small groups of children differential exposure to novel items (cheese, fruits) over a prescribed time period of 26 days (experiment 1) or 25 days (experiment 2). In each study the methods used were essentially the same. The children were subsequently asked to taste pairs of foods and to choose which food they would prefer to eat more. Children chose more of the foods to which they had been exposed than chance would allow, suggesting that there were exposure effects on preference with the majority of subjects (Birch and Marlin, 1982).

Although one may criticise these studies for their complex design, the artificiality of the context and the limited number of subjects, it is important to include them here as the topic is highly relevant to this review, i.e. looking at food preferences in very young children. The authors, too, note 'Particularly for young children, eating is a social occasion and early exposure to food does not occur in a vacuum . . .' (Birch and Marlin, 1982, p. 359), a comment confirmed by the work of Rozin and colleagues, where very young children between the age of 1 year, 4 months and 5 years were offered a wide range of disgusting, inappropriate and unacceptable items to taste. The youngest children were most likely to eat more disgusting items although the majority rejected most of these items. Nevertheless, the authors conclude that a major feature of food selection is learning what not to eat (Rozin *et al.*, 1986).

Experimental research on children's tastes and food preference is influenced by behavioural psychology and seldom takes a 'cultural' angle, for example by looking at cultural explanations for food choice, such as the preference for sweets. Sweets, however, do have a symbolic value in our society, serving a number of functions (for example Taylor and Kiblinski, 1994; Mayall, 1986). (James's study of confectionery does not fall within the scope of this review, since it was published in 1979 and focused upon an older age group – 11- to 17-year-olds.) However, it should be noted as one of the very few studies to investigate the 'meaning' of sweet-eating by children (James, 1979). Sweets are given instead of toys if women are hard up (Taylor and Koblinski, 1994); they are treated as rewards for good behaviour (Birch, Marlin and Rotter, 1984) and as presents from visitors (Mayall, 1986).

The studies reported above suggest that taste is learned at an early age by children. Young children therefore present themselves as an important target group for health interventions which aim to create positive eating habits. Although the experimental studies are viewed as an important mode of research, more work with greater ecological validity would be useful. If 'culture' is recognised as an important context within which eating choices take place then research which has a strong cultural component (such as ethnographic studies) should be prioritised for future work.

Knowledge

Studies suggest that children even at this age (or certainly the older years within the 1–5 age group) do have some knowledge about 'good' and 'bad' foods (authors' terms) and do grasp the bare essentials of health promotion messages (Gorn and Goldberg, 1982; Anliker *et al.*, 1990; Murphy *et al.*, 1995). Murphy and her colleagues, for example, carried out group interviews with 62 US kindergarten pupils (under school age), in groups of 5 or 6, asking them to discuss words associated with nutrition (for example, asking them to name foods with 'lots of fat', 'how people can become too fat', etc.) (Murphy *et al.*, 1995). The study showed that the young children displayed a good understanding of basic concepts. For example, about half correctly identified that people became fat by 'eating too much', about a third said that exercise was a 'way to get rid of extra fat' and correctly defined the term 'nutrition'. The authors noted two specific problems for the children (and for future researchers in this field); the first was that some words had both a technical *and* a lay meaning, such as the word 'fat' which the children saw as meaning overweight rather than a food group. Secondly, some of the nutritional terms were new and unfamiliar to the young children. The study showed that only a proportion of children correctly identified the terms, and the sample size was not large, but the methodology and the concept behind the study is important and repeatable in a UK context. Guidelines only work if the recipients can understand the messages and the identification of the discrepancy between the meaning of certain terms to young children is one important finding from this study (Murphy *et al.*, 1995).

Middle-class mothers in Mayall's qualitative study also reported having definite views on dental caries and their child's teeth, and were more likely to restrict sugar intake because of the effect on teeth (Mayall, 1986). Mayall argues that mothers try to control sugar intake yet gave their young children sweetened drinks – 28% of her sample had seven or more sugared meals or snacks a day, with class differences operating in the predicted direction. This is similar to the findings from studies of mothers with younger children reported in the previous section, such as that carried out by Morgan *et al.* (1995). Mothers' knowledge and awareness about the importance of restricting sugar intake is an important opportunity upon which to build. Lay nutritional knowledge is not always congruent with official recommendations and a greater understanding of where the differences lie, and the reasoning which lies behind mothers' beliefs (other priorities or lack of understanding) would be an important contribution in this area.

Control and food

One of the 'subtexts' of the literature on young children and eating patterns concerns the issue of control. The topic is complicated, however, and while some studies suggest that parents control their children using food as rewards or punishment (for example Casey and Rozin, 1989) others show that even young children learn to use food in a manipulative manner (Lindberg, Bohlin and Hagekull, 1994).

The control that parents may use to influence their children's eating habits has been studied in different ways in psychological literature (for example Birch *et al.*, 1984; Casey and Rozin, 1989) and in sociological work (Mayall, 1986; Devine and Olson, 1992). Casey and Rozin asked parents about which factors they thought induced changes in their young children's eating habits (Casey and Rozin, 1989). This study had a poor response rate (less than 40%) and a very unrepresentative sample but is reviewed as one of the very few studies which provides some survey data on the topic). The researchers sent a questionnaire to a consecutive sample of 200 parents who had at least one child aged 3 or more using a university-based private paediatric practice (Casey and Rozin, 1989).

The study showed a close correlation between methods seen by the parents as effective in encouraging their child to eat certain foods and those used most frequently. Among the latter group, methods used included 'adults like' (i.e. adults like this food) (89.3% reporting that they used this method sometimes or often), 'parents happy' (when the child eats it) (74.4%), 'help prepare' (child helps to prepare food) (72.4%), 'good for you' (food is good for you) (58.6%), and 'reward for eating' (55.3%). The lowest scores were for 'threaten' (if you do not eat this food) (30.5%), 'using as a reward' (23.7%) and 'only food offered' (11.8%) (Casey and Rozin, 1989). The study contained a group biased towards the higher socioeconomic classes which is likely to have influenced the types of responses used (reward rather than punishment) and is based on parents' report rather than practice. Nevertheless, this study is concerned with an important area in dietary change. The findings suggest that positive rather than negative responses on the part of the parents are perceived to be more effective for behaviour change.

The nature of this 'punishment and reward', or social bargaining with children has been explored in some detail (for example by Birch, Marlin and Rotter, 1984). Birch and her colleagues investigated the effects of instrumental eating on food preferences with a group of 45 children (median age 4.2 years). The researchers found, through a complicated experiment, that instrumental consumption of the beverages produced negative shifts in preference; that is, beverages presented as 'means' to other ends were ones that were usually disliked. The group sizes were very small and the study complex; nevertheless, the findings (which have been replicated subsequently) are significant to the review. They imply that the preference for certain foods (for example, vegetables) may acquire negative connotations when they become contingencies; the authors report anecdotal evidence of another study where similar aged children who were told 'Eat your cookies and then you can have your vegetables' burst out laughing (Birch *et al.*, 1984), the request not being consistent with the usual means–end functions of these foods.

While the above research suggests that parents may exercise control over their child's eating habits, other work, both experimental (Lindberg, Bohlin and Hagekull, 1994) and also based upon parents' reports (Mayall, 1986), suggests that children in turn may exert some control over food choice. Mayall only hints at control issues when discussing problems of keeping children happy when shopping, for example, by giving them sweets (Mayall, 1986).

Food refusal, a term without clear definition but involving the 'phenomenon of refusal to eat', is a concept investigated by a number of researchers (for example Lindberg *et al.*, 1994; Birch *et al.*, 1987 and many others). Studies have, however, failed to yield conclusive findings, proposing instead that a constellation of early behaviour problems and temperamental difficulties can be identified (Lindberg, Bohlin and Hagekull, 1994). Concern about 'neophobia' (the fear of new foods) has given rise to a number of experiments with very young children to assess their likelihood of trying new foods; although the studies have conflicting findings, some have found that as children grow older they are more likely to experiment with food (Pelchat and Pliner, 1995), while others showing that younger children were more likely to put anything in their mouths (Rozin *et al.*, 1986), including items regarded by adults as disgusting and dangerous.

These studies focus upon issues not often (explicitly) recognised within health education and draw our attention to the finding that food and control may be at the centre of broader family dynamics. The recognition that some foods are used as rewards and others as contingencies is an important finding and one which helps us to understand the barriers facing the public acceptability of some foods (for example, vegetables) in a more positive light.

Control at mealtimes

Several studies allude to problems with controlling children at the table, with the mother 'being the referee' (Dobson *et al.*, 1994; Mayall, 1986; Seagren and Terry, 1991; Devine and Olson, 1992; Koivisto, Fellenius and Sjøden, 1994; Reed, 1996). These studies, using a variety of methods (for example focus groups, surveys, videoing family mealtimes, interviews) note that mealtimes can become a forum for family tension and stress, with mothers spending more time 'keeping the peace' than being concerned that children ate their food. Devine and Olson, in a US study which drew upon interviews with 36 women, carried out a qualitative analysis of a mother's domestic roles. The authors defined one role for women with young children as the 'peace-keeping role', which involved prevention of family conflicts about food (Devine and Olson, 1992).

Further research from the US provides a different kind of evidence about the food intake of young children and the mothers' reported control (Seagren and Terry, 1991). In this US study, questionnaires were completed by predominantly white female parents of 130 normal weight and 48 obese 3- and 4-year-old children enrolled in a food intervention programme. In the self-reported questionnaires mothers stated that they controlled many aspects of their children's eating including time, frequency and type of food eaten; however, many mothers did not seem to control the amount of food eaten. Although the mothers reported controlling the location of the meal, control was exerted less frequently over snacking while watching television. In four significant ways mothers with children of normal weight differed in their responses to mothers with obese children; differences were that mothers of obese children seemed to control the type of food they allowed their children to eat for snacks less frequently and were less likely to encourage their children to eat all of the food on their plate or to eat as much food as they liked; mothers with normal weight children tended to allow their children to have sweets only after having eaten a good meal more often than the mothers of obese children (Seagren and Terry, 1991).

The findings of both these very different kinds of studies can only be suggestive. However, they both extend our understanding of the importance of the social context of eating habits, and emphasise the point that control over eating is not a simple issue. Seagren and Terry's research provides indirect evidence about the extent of control that some children appear to have in what they eat even at this young age. The link between obesity and control is also implied in the latter study, suggesting that mothers who supervise the food intake more closely may be providing an opportunity for the child to develop good nutritional behaviour.

Research on young children and their eating behaviours and attitudes derives from a range of methods and assumptions although with a notable lack of qualitative studies of parents of young children. The large number of laboratory studies and questionnaire-based studies further emphasises the artificiality of the research situation contrasted with the domestic environment of the young child. Nevertheless, the studies have focused upon issues which are central to this review, namely investigating why children develop preferences for certain foods and not others. For interventions for dietary change to be successful, knowledge about children's preferences and the various influences upon children's eating habits must be developed.

There is some research which suggests that access factors are important, as they were with the other age groups. Nevertheless, the finding that some children living in material hardship will still refuse to eat foods that they do not like suggests a range of cultural factors that are also highly influential. The substantial American literature on the influence of television is not conclusive, and is too culturally specific to be truly applicable to the UK but the research recognises the potentially powerful nature of advertising even at this early age.

Family research, albeit mainly laboratory based, highlights the influence of the young child on decisions about food choice, with children in some families learning early on that they can influence the range of foods they eat. This is a highly significant finding for the review, for attempts at dietary change should be aimed not only at the main carer(s) in the family but should include even young children.

3. Trends for future nutritional health

There is some evidence that household composition is changing and this will have implications for the nutritional patterns of both women and children (and men). Evidence has been presented to suggest that meal composition is dependent upon the dynamics of the household and not simply the food preferences and choices of those directly involved in meal preparation. As fewer women live in nuclear families (with a partner and children), women may, in the future, give their food preferences greater priority than has always occurred in the past.

There are two trends which may modify this possibility. First, more women are now contributing to the paid labour force and, although evidence from the UK is very limited, there is the suggestion that as women spend less time in the home, others (for example, the partner) may become more involved with meal preparation. There are further implications concerned with cooking skills, the extent to which pre-prepared foods may be increasingly used in the home, and the composition of meals. The nutritional benefits or disadvantages of these trends have been little analysed at present. This is also true of the social and cultural impact. Nevertheless, studies have provided evidence that women traditionally attend to family meals, and think about meal composition and the relative merits of different foods, whether or not they always have the opportunity to act on this knowledge. There is no information provided here as to whether others taking over the food preparation role would do likewise.

The second 'trend', of which there is ample evidence at present, is of the continuing material deprivation of many women-headed households. Research has shown clearly that healthy eating is constrained by lack of resources. Greater opportunities for women to join the labour market ease the economic problems for women but in so doing may change the domestic situation so that control of the family's eating patterns is devolved to others.

4. Summary of main findings

Women of childbearing age

The emphasis in the literature is upon the problems rather than the opportunities of access; because of ease of transport, middle-class women have greater opportunities of access to superstores with a wide range of foods; cost is of less importance and storage is not a problem so food can be purchased in bulk.

Most of the literature concentrates upon the barriers to good nutritional practices of women living in conditions of material deprivation where access, cost and storage are all problems. Studies of food availability and cost across neighbourhoods in the UK have emphasised that considerable variation does exist, with better provision available to middle-class neighbourhoods.

Women who live in material deprivation are shown to adopt 'safe' food purchasing strategies which nutritionally may be seen as barriers to healthy eating as they inhibit purchasing of a greater range of foods.

Purchasing of certain foods is not only constrained by cost; research shows that attitudes to certain foods (for example, some vegetables) contribute to a narrow diet and ways of creating greater familiarity with other reasonable-cost foods may form a useful intervention.

One barrier to home cooking is the variety of dry ingredients required to cook and the need for cooking equipment as well as cooking skills. Home cooking interventions need to be tailored to show women how to prepare recipes to suit the available equipment and to reduce recipes to few ingredients.

It may be useful to target interventions relating to dietary change not only at women but also at the males of the household; future trends in the division of labour (for example, through more women working outside the home) may lead to males in the household being more likely to be allocated a major role in food preparation and home cooking.

Given the projections for greater participation by women in the labour market the workplace should be seen as an increasingly significant source of women's nutritional intake in the future and an important venue for nutritional interventions.

At present there is insufficient literature on the topic of eating out and eating fast foods, although in themselves they constitute neither an opportunity nor a barrier. At present there is evidence that the types of food which are 'eaten out' especially by young women (and men) tend to be less nutritious; nevertheless, the opportunity factor to change dietary behaviour in relation to the popular activity of 'eating out' is considerable.

The literature highlights the extent to which food choices privilege male partners and children and that meal composition is decided by all family members (including small children); interventions regarding healthy eating should therefore also be aimed at male partners and children in the family.

Although there is little research on the topic it is evident that snacking is a form of food consumption popular with particular groups (for example, adolescents). The potential for dietary change should be recognised; at present snacking involves less nutritious groups of foods but the range of 'snacks' could be broadened.

The importance of a 'proper meal' is an opportunity to provide families with a variety of vegetables along with other food groups.

Interest in vegetarianism is apparent in young women and men and is linked to an interest in 'health'.

When investigating dietary change it is important not to isolate and focus upon specific nutritional changes but to understand that beliefs and attitudes towards certain foods may belong to broader 'cultural packages'.

Pregnant women

The majority of studies of pregnant women derived from the disciplines included in the search have not looked at the dietary aspects of pregnancy.

Women see pregnancy as an opportunity for dietary change. Interventions could build upon this by targeting women in early pregnancy to encourage dietary change.

Many women are receptive to professional advice in pregnancy and the increased contact which women have with health professionals during pregnancy creates a period of opportunity for professionals.

Many professionals have some general knowledge about nutritional issues in pregnancy but lack specific knowledge especially in relation to folate. More training in nutrition among professional groups (midwives, nursing staff, dietitians) which have high contact with women would be a useful intervention.

Women's knowledge of specific nutritional issues, especially the role of folate early in pregnancy is evident.

Infants under 1

There is a large literature on breastfeeding which is predominantly quantitative and in which women's personal experiences and problems are seldom articulated 'in their own voice'.

Breastfeeding rates have not changed over a ten-year period (1980–1990) and much of the literature does not provide evidence to facilitate an improvement in rates.

Hospital practices are important influences and have introduced a number of changes to encourage breastfeeding. The literature highlights the variation in hospital practices which still exists and the variation in staff attitudes towards the value of breastfeeding. More attention should be directed towards nursing and midwifery staff to understand why these views are still held.

The literature emphasises the finding that breastfeeding is practised more by middle-class, older, better educated mothers who hold more positive attitudes to the practice. Barriers to successful breastfeeding are more likely to be cultural than practical although many women report practical problems in establishing and maintaining breastfeeding.

Interventions could be designed to change the negative views about breastfeeding in public places held by the 'general public'.

Many women wean their children earlier than official recommendations; little research exists which investigates the social and cultural attitudes towards weaning.

Mothers are thoughtful about the diet of their infants; this should form a positive basis for further education. Mothers do not necessarily understand the underlying nutritional messages regarding an infant's diet and the literature documents many examples of infants being fed inappropriate foods for their age.

Professional help is not always seen as appropriate. Different forms of professional interventions may be tried which might increase the legitimacy of the advice for some mothers.

Children aged 1–5 years

There is evidence that children's food choices can be influenced by changing the food messages shown on television and the *potential* for change should make children's television an important forum for future interventions.

Tastes are learnt at an early age. Young children therefore are an important target group for health interventions which help create positive eating habits. However, young children do not always understand food messages in the way that they are intended (for example, the meaning of the term fat).

Lay nutritional knowledge is not always congruent with official recommendations and more understanding of mothers' beliefs is important.

With young children opportunities lie in the identification of positive rewards with eating, but conversely problems may arise when food is used as a means of control.

Mothers who supervise food intake more closely may be providing an opportunity for the child to develop good nutritional behaviour.

5. Recommendations for future research

General areas

The review has identified a number of gaps in the research literature and areas which require more research.

Little research combines investigation of food consumption with attitudes towards nutrition; research tends to examine food consumption or attitudes and beliefs. Closer linkage of consumption with the social context in which food is consumed would form a stronger base for interventions.

There is a lack of qualitative research across the whole field; this is particularly striking in the field of infant feeding with its extensive quantitative literature.

The majority of studies of nutrition have women as their subjects. While women form the basis of this review one key finding is of men's influence in decision-making about meals. More research on men's attitudes towards good nutritional health would be important for future planning.

The symbolic value of different foods is little studied but is essential when contemplating changing eating habits. 'Snacks' and vegetables would be useful starting points for such research.

Different types of eating patterns (for example, grazing, take-away meals) warrant more investigation in terms of both nutrition and the social context of eating.

The social aspects of eating out have been neglected as an opportunity for dietary changes. Little is known about how choices are made concerning the various factors involved in food choice and the relative importance of each (for example, type of food, context, price).

Little is known about the nutritional value of home cooking. This is an area where social scientists and nutritionists could work together. How much do women understand about the cooking process and what are the nutritional and social advantages of home-cooked foods?

Little is known about the use of convenience foods, except that 'working mothers' appear to use them. Preconceptions about convenience foods, attitudes towards use and perceived appropriateness at meals should be investigated.

Women of childbearing age

Little research from the UK has investigated the division of labour within the home and the contribution of all family members to food shopping, preparation and cooking. With women's increasing involvement in the paid labour market this area of research should be given priority.

Although family dynamics in decision-making about food choice within the home may be difficult to study, decision-making within families about meal choice is of considerable significance when considering dietary change. Qualitative methods would be most appropriate in this area of research.

Given the growing importance of the workplace for women more research is required which focuses upon: (a) workplace food (cost, choice, quality), (b) breastfeeding facilities, (c) attitudes of employers to infant feeding, (d) practical approaches to encouragement of breastfeeding mothers in the workplace.

Single women with no dependants remain a neglected group; their nutritional status, eating patterns and food consumption are virtually unknown.

Pregnant women

Although the term 'pre-pregnancy' is used in the medical literature, it is not clear whether it has any meaning for women themselves or to the health professionals who care for them. This could be investigated in further research. Pre-pregnancy can only be seen as an opportunity if the concept has meaning outside the medical field.

Infants under 1

Successful breastfeeding has been little researched. Although factors which identify breast feeders have been identified (for example, past experience, social class, older mothers) little is known beyond this. A more qualitative approach would enable women to report from their own experiences and to identify the barriers to continued breastfeeding.

Although research acknowledges the importance of the Baby Friendly Hospital Initiative there have been few rigorous evaluations of this initiative in the UK literature.

Greater understanding is needed of lay and professional knowledge and understanding of diet, particularly in relation to pregnancy. Research has suggested that there may be differences between lay people and health professionals but these have not been explored.

Children aged 1–5 years

Very little research has explored the role of children in food purchasing; research is required to cover all aspects of this area from the practical side (transport, access) to the preferences which young children may express in relation to certain foods.

The nutritional provision for infants and young children outside the home is a neglected area. For example, a study of the provision by crèches, day-care centres and other carers would be useful. It would be important to examine the congruence and conflicts with parental eating habits.

Most research on influences from the media on children's food choices has been carried out in the US and more UK research is needed; in the UK there may be different patterns of television viewing and different approaches from commercial advertisers. These need to be explored.

Appendices

Appendix A. Summary of studies reviewed in text

Anderson (1991)
Aberdeen, Scotland

Purpose
Explanatory and descriptive

Design
Study type: Cross-sectional + RCT
Data type: Quantitative
Data collection method: Food diaries, interviews
Sample type: Quota and random
Sample size:
Response rate:
Date study carried out:

Comments
PhD thesis
4 studies, 3 descriptive and one experimental

Anderson and Hunt (1992)
West of Scotland

Purpose
Descriptive

Design
Study type: Longitudinal
Data type: Quantitative
Data collection method: Interview and self-completion questionnaires
Sample type: Random
Sample size: 510 females, 443 males
Response rate: 89.9%
Date study carried out: NK

Anderson, Campbell and Shepherd (1993)
Aberdeen, Scotland

Purpose
Descriptive

Design
Study type: Cross-sectional
Data type: Quantitative
Data collection method: Questionnaires + diet diaries, 2 weekdays, 2 weekends
Sample type: Opportunistic (pregnant women), non-pregnant women, matched sample
Sample size: 95 pregnant women
94 non-pregnant women
95/100 pregnant women
94 /100 non-pregnant women
Response rate: NK

Comments
Sample of pregnant women matched for age and area of residence (using postcode) with non-pregnant women

Anderson, Macintyre and West (1993)
West of Scotland

Purpose
Descriptive

Design
Study type: Longitudinal study
Data type: Quantitative
Data collection method: Interviews – semi-structured + self-administered FFQ
Sample type: Stratified random sample
Sample size: 1009 (527 females, 482 males)
Response rate: 86%
Date study carried out: NK

Comments
Study part of West of Scotland Twenty-07 Study: Health in the Community.
917 completed the food frequency questionnaire

Anderson *et al.* (1994a)
5 areas in Scotland

Purpose
Descriptive

Design
Study type: Cross-sectional
Data type: Qualitative and quantitative
Data collection method: Focus and questionnaire
Sample type: Focus groups: quota, questionnaires: quota
Sample size: 8 groups x 8 adults, 1011 adults (questionnaire)
Response rate: NK
Date study carried out: 1992

Anderson, Macintyre and West (1994)
West of Scotland

Purpose
Descriptive

Design
Study type: Longitudinal
Data type: Quantitative
Data collection method: 2 face-to-face interviews + one self-completed questionnaire
Sample type: 2-stage random sample clustered design
Sample size: 1009
Response rate: ?50%
Date study carried out: 1987

Comments
Study part of West of Scotland Twenty-07 Study: Health in the Community
Sample compared to 35-year-old cohort in same study

Anderson *et al.* (1994b)
West of Scotland

Purpose
Descriptive

Design
Study type: Longitudinal
Data type: Quantitative
Data collection method: Face-to-face interview + self-completion questionnaire
Sample type: 2-stage clustered random sample
Sample size: 1710, 852 adults aged 39–40
858 adults aged 59–60
Response rate: NK
Date study carried out: NK

Comments
Study part of West of Scotland Twenty-07 Study: Health in the Community

---

Anderson, Campbell and Shepherd (1995)
Aberdeen, Scotland

Purpose
Explanatory experimental

Design
Study type: RCT
Data type: Quantitative
Data collection method: Questionnaire: self-completion +4-day diet
Sample type: Random
Sample size: 328 women (164 in each group)
Response rate: 5 women refused to take part
Date study carried out: Nov 1987– October 1988

Comments
Study had 3 stages:
1. development of materials
2. development of measures
3. RCT
Sample: pregnant women attending antenatal classes

Anliker et al. (1990)
Western Massachusetts, US

Purpose
Descriptive

Design
Study type: Longitudinal
Data type: Quantitative and quant
Data collection method: Interview, open-ended (children) + (mothers) questionnaire
Sample type: NK
Sample size: 104 children and mothers
Response rate: NK
Date study carried out: NK

Comments
Data from longitudinal Western Massachusetts Growth Study
Sample: 100% white middle upper income families, children aged between 3 years 5 $^1/_2$ months to 3 years 9 $^1/_2$ months: children had open-ended interview + photographs + role-playing

---

Auerbach (1984)
US

Purpose
Descriptive

Design
Study type: Cross-sectional
Data type: Quantitative
Data collection method: Self-completion questionnaire
Sample type: Opportunistic
Sample size: 567
Response rate: 86%
Date study carried out: 1992

Comments
Request for participation sent to 5 journals/women's magazines

---

Backett (1990)
Edinburgh, Scotland

Purpose
Descriptive

Design
Study type: Cross-sectional
Data type: Qualitative
Data collection method: Interviews
Sample type: Random

Sample size: 28 couples each with 2 children
Response rate: NK
Date study carried out: 1987–1988

Comments
4 interviews over 18-month fieldwork period, couples all home-owners with one or both spouses in non-manual occupations

---

Backett (1992)
Edinburgh, Scotland

Purpose
Descriptive

Design
Study type: Cross-sectional
Data type: Qualitative
Data collection method: Interviews
Sample type: Random
Sample size: 28 couples each with 2 children
Response rate: NK
Date study carried out: 1987–1988

Baisch, Fox and Goldberg (1989)
US

Purpose
Descriptive

Design
Study type: Cross-sectional
Data type: Quantitative
Data collection method: Self-completion questionnaire
Sample type: ?Opportunistic
Sample size: 128
Response rate: NK
Date study carried out:

Comments
Study sample are low-income, pregnant adolescents from Teen Pregnancy Service Program

---

Beardsworth and Keil (1991)
UK

Purpose
Descriptive

Design
Study type: Cross-sectional
Data type: Qualitative
Data collection method: Interviews – semi-structured
Sample type: Snowball
Sample size: 76
Response rate: NK
Date study carried out: October 1987–February 1989

Comments
Sample composed of 'self-defined' vegetarians, over the age of 16 and not from religious or ethnic backgrounds where vegetarianisn culturally prescribed

---

Beardsworth and Keil (1993)
UK

Purpose
Descriptive

Design
Study type: Cross-sectional
Data type: Qualitative
Data collection method: Interviews – semi-structured
Sample type: Snowball
Sample size: 76
Response rate: NK
Date study carried out: October 1987–February 1989

Comments
Sample composed of 'self-defined' vegetarians; over the age of 16 and not from religious or ethnic backgrounds where vegetarianism culturally prescribed

---

Becker (1992)
Ireland

Purpose
Descriptive

Design
Study type: Cross-sectional
Data type: Quantitative
Data collection method: Interviews – closed, plus hospital records + postal questionnaire
Sample type: Opportunistic
Sample size: 88 staff
Response rate: 82%
Date study carried out: Spring and summer 1990

Comments
Three maternity units took part, staff sample composed of 76 midwives, 9 obstetric medical staff, three consultant paediatricians

---

Beeken and Waterston (1992)
Newcastle upon Tyne, England

Purpose
Descriptive

Design
Study type: Cross-sectional
Data type: Quantitative
Data collection method: Postal questionnaires for health workers + questionnaire to mothers
Sample type: Opportunistic
Sample size: 197 health workers, 50 mothers

Response rate: 92% staff + 55% mothers
Date study carried out: 1990

Comments
Staff sample composed of hospital and community midwives and health visitors

---

Bergevin, Dougherty and Kramer (1983)
Canada

Purpose
Explanatory

Design
Study type: RCT
Data type: Quantitative
Data collection method: Interviews – closed
Sample type: Opportunistic then random
Sample size: 444
Response rate: NK
Date study carried out: NK

Comments
8.6% could not be reached, none refused to take part
Women excluded if they had twins, the infant died or woman not breastfeeding on discharge

---

Bergman *et al.* (1993)
Gothenberg, Sweden

Purpose
Descriptive

Design
Study type: Cross-sectional
Data type: Quantitative
Data collection method: Questionnaire
Sample type: Opportunistic
Sample size: 133 health professionals
Response rate: NK
Date study carried out: NK

Comments
Sample were working in different health settings – staff samples were midwives and nurses

---

Best, Little and McPherson (1989)
Nottingham, England

Purpose
Descriptive

Design
Study type: Cross-sectional
Data type: Quantitative
Data collection method: Self-completed questionnaires medical records
Sample type: Opportunistic
Sample size: 258
Response rate: 95%
Date study carried out: NK

Birch and Marlin (1982)
Illinois, US

Purpose
Explanatory

Design
Study type: Experimental
Data type: Quantitative
Data collection method: Observational
Sample type: Opportunistic
Sample size: Experiment 1–6 children
Experiment 2–8 children
Response rate: NK
Date study carried out: NK

Comments
Children aged 2 years old;
2 experiments in which children exposed to various foods in experimental situation

---

Birch, Marlin and Rotter (1984)
Illinois, US

Purpose
Explanatory

Design
Study type: Experimental
Data type: Quantitative
Data collection method: Observational
Sample type: Opportunistic
Sample size: 45 (20 males, 25 females)
Response rate: 45 out of 60
Date study carried out: NK

Comments
Median age of children 4.2 years, children assigned to instrumental or control condition

---

Birch *et al.* (1987)
Illinois, US

Purpose
Explanatory

Design
Study type: Experimental
Data type: Quantitative
Data collection method: Observation
Sample type: Opportunistic
Sample size: 43 children
Response rate: 43/58
Date study carried out: NK

Comments
3 age groups of children included:
10 children aged 23–30 months
15 children, 32–42 months, 18 children, 56–69 months
15 children eliminated from study because they failed to meet criteria (either due to illness and missed exposure trials or to failure to look and taste)

Birch *et al.* (1991)
Illinois, US

Purpose
Explanatory

Design
Study type: Experimental
Data type: Quantitative
Data collection method: 24-hour food intake
Sample type: Opportunistic
Sample size: 15 pre-school children
7 boys, 8 girls
Response rate: 100%
Date study carried out: NK

Comments
Sample had a 24-hour food intake measured on 6 days
Sample of 15 children aged 2–5 years attending a day-care centre which served middle-class families

---

Blair and Lichter (1991)
US

Purpose
Descriptive

Design
Study type: Cross-sectional
Data type: Quantitative
Data collection method: Self-completed questionnaires
Sample type: 'weighed representative'
Sample size: 3502
Response rate: NK
Date study carried out: 1988

Comments
Three forms of data collection with varying response rates for each – anthropometric measures for 7414 and self-completion for 6572

Blaxter (1990)
UK

Purpose
Descriptive

Design
Study type: Cross-sectional
Data type: Quantitative and qualitative
Data collection method: Interviews: semi-structured + anthropometric measures + self-completion questionnaire
Sample type: 'Representative of general population'
Sample size: 9003
Response rate: 73.5%
Date study carried out: Autumn 1984–summer 1985

Comments
Three forms of data collection;
interviews, part open-ended,
nurse visit + anthropometric measures
self-completion questionnaire

Bloom *et al.* (1982)
Halifax, Nova Scotia

Purpose
descriptive

Design
Study type: Cross-sectional
Data type: Quantitative
Data collection method: Interview – closed
Sample type: Not specified
Sample size: 539 mothers
Response rate: 100%
Date study carried out: NK

Comments
Excluded from study were mothers of twins or infants weighing less than 2500 grams or having Apgar score of less than 5, those women relinquishing their infant or those who did not speak or understand English

---

Bruce, Khan and Olsen (1991)
London, England

Purpose
Descriptive

Design
Study type: Cross-sectional
Data type: Quantitative
Data collection method: Midwives, self-completed questionnaire; mothers, interview closed, 2 days postpartum + postal questionnaire
Sample type: Opportunistic
Sample size: 60 staff, 202 mothers
Response rate: 80% staff, 81.2% mothers (postal)
Date study carried out: 1988

Bruce and Griffioen (1995)
London, England

Purpose
Descriptive

Design
Study type: Cross-sectional
Data type: Quantitative
Data collection method: Midwives – self-completed questionnaire; women, postal questionnaire at 6 weeks

Sample type: Opportunistic
Sample size: 65 staff, 322 mothers
Response rate: 87% staff, 80% mothers
Date study carried out: 1990

Cade and Booth (1990)
3 English towns

Purpose
Descriptive

Design
Study type: Cross-sectional
Data type: Quantitative
Data collection method: 24-hour dietary record
Sample type: Stratified random sample
Sample size: 1115 men,1225 women
Response rate: 85%
Date study carried out: NK

Comments
If subjects did not complete dietary record, interviewer took 24-hour recall of food intake for previous day

---

Calnan (1990)
South-East England

Purpose
Descriptive

Design
Study type: Cross-sectional
Data type: Qualitative
Data collection method: Interview
Sample type: Opportunistic
Sample size: 21 women social class I and II
16 women social class IV and V
Response rate: NK
Date study carried out: 1986

Comments
Sample white women aged 20–35 years with at least one adult in household working, living as married or married

---

Carty and Bradley (1990)
Vancouver, Canada

Purpose
Explanatory

Design
Study type: RCT
Data type: Quantitative
Data collection method: Questionnaires, nurses' assessments
Sample type: Opportunistic, then randomly assigned to different discharge times
Sample size: 131
Response rate: NK
Date study carried out: NK

Comments
Women randomised to one of three postpartum discharge times.
Criteria of eligibility not detailed. Questionnaires left with women on four occasions at 37 weeks pregnancy, during hospital stay, 1 week and 1 month postpartum

---

Casey and Rozin (1989)
US

Purpose
Descriptive

Design
Study type: Cross-sectional
Data type: Quantitative
Data collection method: Self-completion questionnaires
Sample type: Opportunistic
Sample size: 200
Response rate: 76
Date study carried out: NK

Comments
Parents sampled from university-based private paediatric practice, with one child aged 3 years or more

---

Chalmers (1991)
Edinburgh, Scotland

Purpose
Descriptive

Design
Study type: Cross-sectional
Data type: Quantitative
Data collection method: Telephone interviews
Sample type: Random sample
Sample size: 40
Response rate: NK
Date study carried out: NK

Comments
Sample of 9 community midwives and 31 health visitors

Charles and Kerr (1988)
York, England

Purpose
Descriptive

Design
Study type: Cross-sectional
Data type: Qualitative and quantitative
Data collection method: Interviews with open-ended questions, 2-week food diary
Sample type: Opportunistic
Sample size: 200 women with at least one child under school age
Response rate: NK
Date study carried out: 1982–1983

Comments
Women interviewed twice with gap of two weeks during which time they completed the food diary for everyone in household
181 women interviewed on the first occasion, 157 women completed food diaries

---

Clark and Fisk (1994)
England

Purpose
Descriptive

Design
Study type: Cross-sectional
Data type: Quantitative
Data collection method: Interview – closed
Sample type: Opportunistic
Sample size: 417
Response rate: NK
Date study carried out: NK

Cornelius (1991)
US

Purpose
Descriptive

Design
Study type: Cross-sectional
Data type: Quantitative
Data collection method: Structured questionnaire
Sample type: National multi-stage probability sample
Sample size: 6722 children 5–17 years
Response rate: Cumulative response rate 79.7%
Date study carried out: 1 Jan–31 December 1987

Comments
Data from 1987 National Medical Expenditure Survey of approximately 15 000 households:
4 face-to-face interviews + 1 telephone interview
Blacks, Hispanics, elderly, functionally impaired over-sampled

---

Cotugna *et al.* (1992)
US

Purpose
Descriptive

Design
Study type: Cross-sectional
Data type: Quantitative
Data collection method: Questionnaire
Sample type: National probability sample
Sample size: 22 043
Response rate: NK
Date study carried out: 1987

Comments
Data part of a larger study:
Cancer Control Supplement of 1987
National Health Interview Survey with 22 043 adults aged 18–99

Cox *et al.* (1996)
UK

Purpose
Descriptive

Design
Study type: Cross-sectional
Data type: Quantitative
Data collection method: Questionnaires – structured
Sample type: Stratified random
Sample size: 741 adults
Response rate: NK
Date study carried out: NK

Comments
Sample to reflect regional and social class profile of the UK

Crotty, Rutishauser and Cahill (1992)
Australia

Purpose
Descriptive

Design
Study type: Cross-sectional
Data type: Qualitative and quantitative
Data collection method: 3-day food diaries + interviews – open-ended, plus single 3-day weighed food record
Sample type: Opportunistic
Sample size: 29
Response rate: 29/36
Date study carried out: NK

Comments
Study sample very small and with the different forms of data gathering, a high-drop out rate

---

Dawson, Jeffrey and Walsh (1988)
North-western US

Purpose
Explanatory

Design
Study type: Experimental
Data type: Quantitative
Data collection method: Observation
Sample type: Opportunistic then random
Sample size: 80 school pupils
Response rate: 94% permission forms returned
Date study carried out: NK

Comments
Sample white, middle-class, public school kindergarten students

Mean age 6.2 years.
Children randomly assigned to one of eight conditions

Devine and Olson (1992)
NY State, US

Purpose
Descriptive

Design
Study type: Cross-sectional
Data type: Qualitative
Data collection method: Interviews
Sample type: Purposive
Sample size: 36 women
Response rate: NK
Date study carried out:

Comments
Women sampled from three life stages:
14 aged 32–43
10 aged 38–46
12 aged 46–63

Dittus, Hillers and Beerman (1995)
Washington State, US

Purpose
Descriptive

Design
Study type: Cross-sectional
Data type: Quantitative
Data collection method: Postal questionnaire
Sample type: Random
Sample size: 1069
Response rate: 60%
Date study carried out: 1990

Comments
Qualitative pilot study and focus groups

Dobson *et al.* (1994)
England

Purpose
Descriptive

Design
Study type: Cross-sectional
Data type: Qualitative and quantitative
Data collection method: Individual and group interviews food expenditure diaries and consumption diaries
Sample type: Non-random – see Comments
Sample size: 48 families
Response rate: NK
Date study carried out:

Comments
Half the sample were lone parents, half were two-parent families
Sample were selected to 'ensure that a range of different situations and experiences could be investigated'; 2 contrasting areas of the city were chosen, all families were receiving Income Support except 4 which were slightly over the IS threshold

---

Douthitt (1989)
Canada

Purpose
Descriptive

Design
Study type: Cross-sectional
Data type: Quantitative
Data collection method: Telephone interview – closed
Sample type: Random
Sample size: 429 married women
437 married men
Response rate: NK
Date study carried out: 1981

Comments
Data from National Time Budget Sample using sample which omitted households with more than three adults
Adults aged 15 years and over

Dowler and Calvert (1995)
Greater London, England

Purpose
Descriptive

Design
Study type: Cross-sectional
Data type: Quantitative and qualitative
Data collection method: Semi-structured interviews, food frequency questionnaire, 3-day dietary intake record
Sample size: Random
Sample type: Minimum data on 200 households
Response rate: NK
Date study carried out: May 1992–June 1993

Comments
Study of lone parents sampled in a variety of stages

Doyle *et al.* (1982)
London, England

Purpose
Descriptive

Design
Study type: Cross-sectional
Data type: Quantitative
Data collection method: 7-day weighed diet records, plus blood samples
Sample size: Opportunistic
Sample type: 71 mothers
Response rate: 71/76

Date study carried out: NK

Comments
Mothers recruited from Salvation Army Mothers Hospital

Drake (1992)
Kansas City, Missouri, US

Purpose
Descriptive

Design
Study type: Cross-sectional
Data type: Quantitative and qualitative
Data collection method: Food diary + interview, food intake diary, anthropometric measures + biochemical
Sample type: Opportunistic
Sample size: 96
Response rate: 96/126
Date study carried out: January 1989–January 1990

Dusdieker *et al.* (1985)
Iowa City, Iowa, US

Purpose
Descriptive

Design
Study type: Cross-sectional
Data type: Quantitative
Data collection method: Questionnaires (structured)
Sample type: Opportunistic
Sample size: 94 breastfeeding, 52 bottle feeding mothers
Response rate: 94/100, 54/57 mothers
Date study carried out: NK

Comments
Sample eligible if breast or bottle feeding infant from birth, and if breastfeeding for 6–8 weeks with minimal supplementation
Complete data on all subjects not obtained

Eiser and Eiser (1985)
UK

Purpose
Descriptive

Design
Study type: Cross-sectional
Data type: Quantitative
Data collection method: Interview – closed
Sample type: Opportunistic
Sample size: 48 women
Response rate: NK
Date study carried out: NK

Comments
Sample contacted through GP clinics

Ellis (1983)
British Columbia, Canada

Purpose
Descriptive

Design
Study type: Cross-sectional
Data type: Quantitative
Data collection method: Questionnaire self-completion
Sample type: Opportunistic
Sample size: 408 school pupils
Response rate: NK
Date study carried out: NK

Comments
9 schools participated

Evans, Lyons and Killien (1986)
Seattle, Washington, US

Purpose
Explanatory

Design
Study type: RCT
Data type: Quantitative
Data collection method: Telephone interview
Sample type: Quota then random
Sample size: 95 women (see under Comments)
Response rate: NK
Date study carried out: NK

Comments
Criteria of eligibility included infant in normal nursery, discharged with mother, women breastfeeding on discharge. Randomised sample was 55 mothers in formula group and 40 mothers in no formula group

---

Forsyth, Macintyre and Anderson (1994)
Glasgow, Scotland

Purpose
Descriptive

Design
Study type: Longitudinal
Data type: Quantitative
Data collection method: Interview in respondent's home
Sample type: Two-stage random sample clustered design
Sample size: 691
Response rate: 81% of those originally interviewed in 1987/88
Date study carried out: 1992

Comments
Study part of West of Scotland Twenty-07 Study: Health in the Community
Two older age groups included in this study, resident in the two study localities in 1987/88

Frank *et al.* (1987)
Boston, US

Purpose
Explanatory

Design
Study type: RCT
Data type: Quantitative
Data collection method: Structured interview, telephone structured interview, 24-hour dietary recall of infant feeding practices
Sample type: Opportunistic, then randomisation
Sample size: 343
Response rate: 83%
Date study carried out: May 1984 to September 1985

Comments
Selection criteria: women having breastfed at least once in hospital, English or Spanish speaking, telephone in home, infant not requiring more than 48 hours in NICU.
Two interventions, breastfeeding counselling and discharge pack.
Of those recruited 8% refused to take part and 9% were missed

Freed and Fraley (1993)
Houston, Texas, US

Purpose
Descriptive

Design
Study type: Cross-sectional
Data type: Quantitative
Data collection method: Self-completed questionnaires
Sample type: Opportunistic
Sample size: 268 expectant mothers
Response rate: NK
Date study carried out: NK

Comments
Mothers sampled from childbirth preparation classes at 5 private hospitals

Fuller and Mackie (1996)
Greater Manchester, England

Purpose
Descriptive

Design
Study type: Cross-sectional
Data type: Qualitative?
Data collection method: Interview
Sample type: Opportunistic
Sample size: 175
Response rate: NK
Date study carried out: NK

Furst *et al.* (1996)
New York, US

Purpose
Descriptive

Design
Study type: Cross-sectional
Data type: Qualitative
Data collection method: Interviews – semi-structured
Sample type: Purposive
Sample size: 29 adults
Response rate: NK
Date study carried out: NK

Comments
Sample primarily middle income, Caucasian

Gabriel, Gabriel and Lawrence (1986)
NY State, US

Purpose
Descriptive

Design
Study type: Cross-sectional
Data type: Quantitative
Data collection method: Interview – closed
Sample type: Opportunistic
Sample size: 313 women
Response rate: 313/317 women
Date study carried out: June–August 1983

Comments
Sample of women with 'normal labour' and 'normal' infant: women interviewed day after delivery

Gibney and Lee (1993)
Dublin, Ireland

Purpose
Descriptive

Design
Study type: Cross-sectional
Data type: Quantitative
Data collection method: 7-day food and nutrition intake history
Sample type: Random
Sample size:
Response rate: 94%
Date study carried out: NK

Goodine and Fried (1982)
Ottowa, Canada

Purpose
Descriptive

Design
Study type: Prospective cohort
Data type: Quantitative
Data collection method: Self-completed questionnaire
Sample size: Opportunistic
Sample type: 288
Response rate: 78%
Date study carried out: NK

Comments
Study uses a sub-sample of women from the Ottowa Prenatal Prospective study: women interviewed in each trimester and sub-sample sent a questionnaire when the infant was one year

---

Gorn and Goldberg (1982)
Quebec, Canada

Purpose
Explanatory

Design
Study type: Experimental
Data type: Quantitative
Data collection method: Observation
Sample size: Random
Sample type: 72 children
Response rate: NK
Date study carried out: NK

Comments
Children at summer camp
juniors = 5–6 years
seniors = 7–8 years
children randomly assigned to each of 2 treatments during each of 2 sessions (n = 288)

Gregg (1989)
Liverpool, England

Purpose
Descriptive

Design
Study type: Cross-sectional
Data type: Quantitative
Data collection method: Self-completion questionnaire
Sample size: Opportunistic
Sample type: 400
Response rate: NK
Date study carried out: NK

Comments
Fourth-form pupils from ten comprehensive schools

Grossman *et al.* (1990)
Columbus, Ohio, US

Purpose
Descriptive

Design
Study type: Cross-sectional
Data type: Quantitative
Data collection method: Medical records + structured interviews postpartum + 8 week telephone interview
Sample size: Opportunistic
Sample type: 220 women
Response rate: 220/235
Date study carried out: NK

Hally *et al.* (1984)
Newcastle upon Tyne, England

Purpose
Descriptive

Design
Study type: Longitudinal
Data type: Quantitative
Data collection method: Interviews (structured), postal questionnaire and medical records
Sample type: Opportunistic
Sample size: 507
Response rate: 86%
Date study carried out: NK

Comments
Sample of women were enrolled into the study over a period of 65 weeks, women were aged at least 16, resident in the city, 34 weeks pregnant and free from illnesses liable to preclude breastfeeding
Women interviewed antenatally, 6 weeks after delivery and postal questionnaire 3 months postpartum

---

Hamilton (1993)
Reading and London, England

Purpose
Descriptive

Design
Study type: Cross-sectional
Data type: Quantitative and qualitative
Data collection method: Questionnaire (Reading)
Interview (festival)
Sample type: 'Quota' sample – Reading
Opportunistic (festival)
Sample size: 304 (Reading), 402 (festival)
Response rate: NK
Date study carried out: 1990

Comments
Samples – 1 from Reading, a 'general population' sample with a range of groups, and a sample from Festival of Mind, Body and Spirit

Haste *et al.* (1990)
London, England

Purpose
Descriptive

Design
Study type: Cross-sectional
Data type: Quantitative
Data collection method: Interview – closed, 28 week and 36 week dietary assessments
Sample type: Random sampling
Sample size: 184
Response rate: 184/288
Date study carried out: August 1982–August 1984

Comments
Sample composed of Caucasian women presenting at hospital antenatal booking clinic, 83 smokers, 101 non-smokers

Health Education Authority (1989)
3 cities in England

Purpose
Descriptive

Design
Study type: Cross-sectional
Data type: Qualitative and quantitative
Data collection method: Two 48-hour food diaries and semi-structured interviews
Sample type: Opportunistic, sometimes snowball sampling
Sample size: 47 households
Response rate: NK
Date study carried out: May to June 1988

Comments
20 one-parent families, 12 two-parent families, 15 single people. All households not more than 20 per cent above the level of Income Support

Holt and Wolkind (1983)
UK

Purpose
Descriptive

Design
Study type: Longitudinal
Data type: Quantitative
Data collection method: Interview – closed antenatally, 4 months and 14 months postpartum
Sample type: Consecutive sample then random sub-sample
Sample size: 106
Response rate: 106/131
Date study carried out: 1974

Comments
Sample of women attending antenatal clinic, orginally screened for possible inclusion in longitudinal study

James (1981)
Manchester, England

Purpose
Descriptive

Design
Study type: Cross-sectional
Data type: Quantitative
Data collection method: Structured interview + case notes, postal questionnaire at 6 months
Sample type: Opportunistic
Sample size: 302
Response rate: 78% of postal questionnaire
Date study carried out: 1978

Comments
Study set up to follow a cohort of British born women and their children

Jeffrey, McLellarn and Fox (1982)
US

Purpose
Explanatory

Design
Study type: Experimental
Data type: Quantitative
Data collection method: Observation + BET and food attitude scale
Sample type: Opportunistic then random
Sample size: 47 children
Response rate: NK
Date study carried out: NK

Comments
Children randomly assigned to three experimental groups. Ages 4–5 years

Jensen, Rao and Hilton (1989)
Arkansas, US

Purpose
Descriptive

Design
Study type: Cross-sectional
Data type: Quantitative
Data collection method: Postal questionnaire
Sample type: 'Representative of state of Arkansas'
Sample size: 310 in 1980, 294 in 1986
Response rate: 1980 87%, 1986 79%
Date study carried out: 1980, 1986

Comments
Data are from the Arkensas Household Research Panel, a survey carried out yearly in the state

Johnson, Smiciklas-Wright and Crouter (1992)
US

Purpose
Descriptive

Design
Study type: Cross-sectional
Data type: Quantitative
Data collection method: Questionnaire + 4 non-consecutive days of dietary intake
Sample type: ?
Sample size: 215 children aged 2–5 years + their mothers
Response rate: 215/250
Date study carried out: 1985

Comments
Data from US Department of Agriculture 1985
Continuing Survey of Food Intakes of Individuals (CSFII)
Target child randomly selected from each family

Jones (1987)
UK

Purpose
Descriptive

Design
Study type: Cross-sectional
Data type: Qualitative and quantitative
Data collection method: Semi-structured interviews
Sample type: Opportunistic
Sample size: 1525
Response rate: 98.7%
Date study carried out: NK

Jones and West (1986)
UK

Purpose
Explanatory

Design
Study type: RCT
Data type: Quantitative
Data collection method: Semi-structured questionnaires at12 months
Sample type: Opportunistic then randomisation
Sample size: 678 in original sample
Response rate: 96%
Date study carried out: NK

Kilcast, Cathro and Morris (1996)
UK

Purpose
Descriptive

Design
Study type: Cross-sectional
Data type: Qualitative and quantitative
Data collection method: Focus groups, interviews + tasks checklist + follow-up interviews + survey
Sample type: Opportunistic
Sample size: NK
Response rate: NK
Date study carried out: NK

Comments
3 stages to study:
depth interviews + focus groups, followed by 'tips brochure and tasks checklist' to low vegetable consumers, then follow-up interviews with these consumers.
Original groups reconvened for discussion and a follow-up survey after a further 5 months

Kim (1989)
Canada

Purpose
Descriptive

Design
Study type: Cross-sectional
Data type: Quantitative
Data collection method: Questionnaire
Sample type: National clustered probability sample
Sample size: 3511
Response rate: NK
Date study carried out: 1982–83

Comments
Sample contains only married women, French or English, the language most often spoken at home, self-employed. full-time or part-time employed or housewife with no paid job. 3511 met the criteria from a larger sample/study

Klesges *et al.* (1990)
Memphis, Tennessee, US

Purpose
Descriptive

Design
Study type: Experimental
Data type: Quantitative
Data collection method: Observation of children, mothers Self-completion questionnaire + height and weight, child + mother
Sample type: Opportunistic
Sample size: 53 (26 male, 27 female)
Response rate: NK
Date study carried out: NK

Comments
Mean age of child 5.3 years; children excluded if adopted, handicapped, with dietary restrictions or allergies, outside age group; sample 98% Caucasian

---

Kogan *et al.* (1994)
48 US states and District of Columbia

Purpose
Explanatory

Design
Study type: Cross-sectional
Data type: Quantitative
Data collection method: Questionnaire to women 6–17 months postnatally – by mail, phone, or personal interview
Sample type: 'Nationally representative'
Sample size: 9924
Response rate: 74% for overall study
Date study carried out: 1988

Comments
Data from 1988 National Maternal and Infant Health Survey, a 'follow-back' study with 3 cohorts
Women included if they had a live birth in 1988

Koivisto, Fellenius and Sjøden (1994)
Uppsala, Sweden

Purpose
Descriptive

Design
Study type: Cross-sectional
Data type: Quantitative
Data collection method: Video-recordings + weighed dietary intake for 7-day period
Sample type: See under Comments
Sample size: 50 families
Response rate: NK
Date study carried out: NK

Comments
Study part of larger study of 599 families randomly selected, from which this sample drawn from volunteers

---

Kotz and Story (1994)
US

Purpose
Descriptive

Design
Study type: Content analysis
Data type: Quantitative
Data collection method: Observational
Sample type:
Sample size:
Response rate:
Date study carried out: October 1991, January, February 1992

Comments
5 TV networks studied 7am to 10am, 3 Saturday mornings. 52.5 hours of children's TV viewing contained 997 food commercials and 68 public service announcements

---

Lilburne *et al.* (1988)
New South Wales, Australia

Purpose
Descriptive

Design
Study type: Cross-sectional
Data type: Quantitative
Data collection method: Questionnaire with 52 items
Sample type: 'Quota'
Sample size: 274 mothers
Response rate: 95%
Date study carried out: NK

Lindberg, Bohlin and Hagekull (1994)
Uppsala, Sweden

Purpose
Experimental

Design
Study type: Experimental/longitudinal
Data type: Quantitative
Data collection method: Mother interviewed on several occasions,plus anthropometric data collected
Sample type: See under Comments
Sample size: 24 in experimental group, 24 in control group
Response rate: NK
Date study carried out:

Comments
Infants recruited through two parent questionnaire population studies and from Child Health Centers (CHCs). 5 inclusion criteria and 3 exclusion criteria left 24 infants in 'experimental' group. Controls were matched for age, sex and CHC affiliation, the latter a proxy for area of living. Data collected over first year of infant's life
j111

London Food Commission (undated)
London, England

Purpose
Descriptive

Design
Study type: Cross-sectional
Data type: Quantitative
Data collection method: Questionnaire
Sample type: NK
Sample size: 17 stores
Response rate: NK

Date study carried out: March 1985

Comments
Shopping price survey;
10 items chosen, supermarkets of different sizes

McIntosh (1985)
Glasgow, Scotland

Purpose
Descriptive

Design
Study type: Longitudinal
Data type: Qualitative
Data collection method: Semi-structured interviews
Sample type: See under Comments
Sample size: 80 first-time mothers
Response rate: NK
Date study carried out: 1981–1982

Comments
Women were interviewed on 6 occasions: 1 time antenatally and 5 postnatal interviews sampled randomly from 3 antenatal clinics but exclusively from social classes III, IV and V

McIntosh (1986)
Glasgow, Scotland

Purpose
Descriptive

Design
Study type: Longitudinal
Data type: Qualitative
Data collection method: Semi-structured interviews
Sample type: Opportunistic
Sample size: 80 first-time mothers
Response rate: NK
Date study carried out: 1981–1982

Comments
Women were interviewed on 6 occasions: 1 time antenatally and 5 postnatal interviews sampled randomly from 3 antenatal clinics but exclusively from social classes III, IV and V

McIntyre (1991)
Nova Scotia

Purpose
Descriptive

Design
Study type: Cross sectional
Data type: Quantitative
Data collection method: Questionnaire – self-completion
Sample type: Schools selected using 'stratified random sample', pupils selected opportunistically
Sample size: 2520 November, 2498 December
Response rate: NK
Date study carried out: November and December 1991

Comments
Study used the Halifax Breakfast Survey (pictorial), data collection repeated to give 2 estimates of breakfast eating; 25 schools from across the province involved in study

---

McIntyre and Horbul (1995)
Northern Ontario, Canada

Purpose
Descriptive

Design
Study type: Cross-sectional
Data type: Quantitative
Data collection method: Self-completion questionnaire
Sample type: Opportunistic
Sample size: 4079
Response rate: NK
Date study carried out: September and December 1993

Comments
Study used the Halifax Breakfast Survey (pictorial), data collection repeated to give 2 estimates of breakfast eating; 50 schools in 15 communities took part in study

---

Mackie, Wood and Gregory (1993)
Cleveland, England

Purpose
Descriptive

Design
Study type: Cross-sectional
Data type: Qualitative
Data collection method: Focus groups
Sample type: Opportunistic
Sample size: 72
Response rate: NK
Date study carried out: 1989

McKillop and Durnin (1982)
Glasgow, Scotland

Purpose
Descriptive

Design
Study type: Cross-sectional
Data type: Quantitative
Data collection method: Food diary + questionnaire + anthropometric measures
Sample type: Quota?
Sample size: 305 children
Response rate: 9 refusals, 215 non-replies

Comments
5-day food diary collected
Children aged between 9 months and 2 years

Maehr *et al.* (1993)
California, US

Purpose
Descriptive

Design
Study type: Cross-sectional
Data type: Quantitative
Data collection method: Interview – closed + medical records
Sample type: Matched sample
Sample size: 48 teen mothers, 48 adult mothers
Response rate: NK
Date study carried out: August–December 1989

Comments
'Teen' defined as 14–18, 'adult' defined as 23–33
Largely Hispanic sample

Manstead, Proffitt and Smart (1983)
Manchester, England

Purpose
Experimental

Design
Study type: Experimental
Data type: Quantitative
Data collection method: Self-completed questionnaires
Sample type: Opportunistic
Sample size: 250 experimental group, 85 control group
Response rate: 85/154 for control group
Date study carried out: NK

Comments
Women recruited from antenatal clinics, mothers were aged between 16 and 40 years and were at least 24 weeks pregnant
Two-stage study, with predictive and follow-up questionnaire; control group recruited later and did not complete the predictive questionnaire

---

Martens and Warde (1997)
UK

Purpose
Descriptive

Design
Study type: Cross-sectional
Data type: Qualitative and quantitative
Data collection method: In-depth interviews and structured interviews
Sample type: Quota
Sample size: 30 (for in-depth study) , 1001 (structured study)
Response rate:
Date study carried out: 1994–1995

Matich and Simms (1992)
Pennsylvania, US

Purpose
Descriptive

Design
Study type: Longitudinal
Data type: Quantitative
Data collection method: Self-completion questionnaire
Sample type: Opportunistic
Sample size: 159
Response rate: 'Approximately' 99%
Date study carried out: June 1985–January 1986

Comments
Questionnaire completed in third trimester of pregnancy. 2nd self-administered questionnaire at 4 weeks postpartum for breastfeeding women only.
Women sampled from prenatal clinics, prenatal classes and WIC clinics

---

Mayall (1986)
Inner London, England

Purpose
Descriptive

Design
Study type: Cross-sectional
Data type: Qualitative
Data collection method: Interviews – semi-structured
Sample type: Opportunistic
Sample size: 135
Response rate: 82%
Date study carried out: 1982

Comments
Sample comprised white mothers, born in British Isles with husband or boyfriend, first child aged 18–36 months.
8% unwilling to take part, 10% moved away before study started

---

Medical Research Council Vitamin Study Research Group (1991)
International

Purpose
Explanatory

Design
Study type: RCT-double blind
Data type: Quantitative
Data collection method: Medical records
Sample type: Opportunistic
Sample size: 1195
Response rate: 1195/1817
Date study carried out: July 1983–April 1991

Comments
33 centres took part, 17 in the UK, 16 in other countries. Women with previous NTD and not taking vitamin supplements eligible for trial

---

Mooney (1990)
London, England

Purpose
Descriptive

Design
Study type: Cross-sectional
Data type: Quantitative
Data collection method: Questionnaire and shopping price questionnaire
Sample type: Opportunistic
Sample size: 9 supermarkets
Response rate: NK
Date study carried out: NK

Comments
4 supermarkets in affluent areas, 5 in deprived areas

Morgan *et al.* (1995)
5 urban and rural areas of England

Purpose
Descriptive

Design
Study type: Cross-sectional
Data type: Quantitative
Data collection method: Semi-structured questionnaire
Sample type: 'Quota'
Sample size: 1004
Response rate: NK
Date study carried out: June –September/October 1992

Comments
Health visitors involved in collecting data from mothers; all mothers enrolled if infant between 3–12 months.
No details of quota sampling provided

Morgan and Stordy (1995)
5 urban and rural areas of England

Purpose
Descriptive

Design
Study type: Cross-sectional
Data type: Quantitative
Data collection method: Semi-structured questionnaires
Sample type: Opportunistic
Sample size: 1004
Response rate: NK
Date study carried out: June –September 1992

Comments
Health visitors involved in collecting data from mothers; all mothers enrolled if infant 3–12 months
No details of quota sampling provided

Mulliner, Spiby and Fraser (1995)
Trent, England

Purpose
Descriptive

Design
Study type: Cross-sectional
Data type: Qualitative
Data collection method: Semi-structured interview
Sample type: Multi-stage random sampling
Sample size: 77
Response rate: 78%
Date study carried out: NK

Murcott (1982)
South Wales

Purpose
Descriptive

Design
Study type: Cross-sectional
Data type: Qualitative
Data collection method: Interview – semi-structured
Sample type: Opportunistic
Sample size: 37
Response rate: NK
Date study carried out: 1979–1980

Murcott (1983)
South Wales

Purpose
Descriptive

Design
Study type: Cross-sectional
Data type: Qualitative
Data collection method: Interview – semi-structured
Sample type: Opportunistic
Sample size: 37
Response rate: NK
Date study carried out: 1979–1980

Murcott (1988)
South Wales

Purpose
Descriptive

Design
Study type: Cross-sectional
Data type: Qualitative
Data collection method: Interview – semi-structured
Sample type: Opportunistic
Sample size: 37
Response rate: NK
Date study carried out: 1979–1980

Murphy *et al.* (1995)
Michigan, US

Purpose
Descriptive

Design
Study type: Cross-sectional
Data type: Qualitative
Data collection method: Focus groups
Sample type: Opportunistic
Sample size: 62
Response rate: NK
Date study carried out: May 1993

Comments
Sample from 2 elementary schools with 12 groups of 'about' 5 students per group

---

Murray et al. (1993)
Grampian, Scotland

Purpose
Descriptive

Design
Study type: Cross-sectional
Data type: Quantitative
Data collection method: Postal questionnaire
Sample type: Opportunistic
Sample size: 58
Response rate: 58/70
Date study carried out: November 1990

Comments
Sample comprises 26 general practitioners, 20 community nurses, 12 practice nurses

---

National Children's Homes (1991)
Scotland to Devon

Purpose
Descriptive

Design
Study type: Cross-sectional
Data type: Qualitative and quantitative
Data collection method: Detailed questionnaire, in-depth interviews
Sample type: Opportunistic
Sample size: 354
Response rate: NK
Date study carried out: January 1991

Comments
Families sampled from 52 NCH homes: 19 families selected for in-depth interview study

---

Neifert *et al.* (1988a)
Denver, Colorado, US

Purpose
Explanatory

Design
Study type: RCT – prospective double blind
Data type: Quantitative
Data collection method: Standardised questionnaire, either given at hospital or by telephone at 2 weeks postpartum, follow-up questionnaire at 2 months or weaning
Sample type: Opportunistic
Sample size: 60 breastfeeding mothers
Response rate: NK
Date study carried out: NK

Comments
Mothers under 18 years of age

Neifert *et al.* (1988b)
Denver, Colorado, US

Purpose
Descriptive

Design
Study type: Cross-sectional
Data type: Quantitative
Data collection method: Questionnaire within 48 hours birth 2 follow-up questionnaires, 2 weeks,2 months
Sample type: Opportunistic
Sample size: 244
Response rate: NK
Date study carried out: 1982–83

Nolan and Goel (1995)
Ontario, Canada

Purpose
Descriptive

Design
Study type: Longitudinal
Data type: Quantitative
Data collection method: Questionnaire
Sample type: Multi-stage stratified cluster for original sample
Sample size: 3120
Response rate: 'Non-response rate 0.67' to breastfeeding question
Date study carried out: 1986–1990

Comments
Sample obtained from the Ontario Health Survey which has two stages: an interviewer-completed questionnaire and a self-completed questionnaire. Data for this paper from the latter

---

Oakley and Rajan (1993)
England

Purpose
Descriptive

Design
Study type: Longitudinal
Data type: Quantitative
Data collection method: Postal questionnaires
Sample type: Opportunistic
Sample size: 362
Response rate: 78% for questionnaire when infant 1 year
95% for questionnaire 6 weeks postpartum
Date study carried out: 1985–1988

Comments
Part of a larger study: Social Support and Pregnancy Outcome Study

---

Olson, Ponzetti and Olson (1989)
11 US states

Purpose
Descriptive

Design
Study type: Cross-sectional
Data type: Quantitative
Data collection method: Time record chart + questionnaire
Sample type: Quota
Sample size: 445
Response rate: NK
Date study carried out:

Comments
Study part of larger study: 11 Interstate Urban/Rural Comparison of Families' Time Use, subsample of 2-parent family household with 2 children, at least one pre-school and one full-time homemaker

---

Pearson *et al.* (1996)
Sheffield, England

Purpose
Descriptive

Design
Study type: Cross-sectional
Data type: Quantitative
Data collection method: Questionnaire
Sample type: Opportunistic
Sample size: 60 women
16 health professionals
Response rate: NK
Date study carried out: NK

Pelchat and Pliner (1995)
Canada

Purpose
Explanatory

Design
Study type: Experimental
Data type: Quantitative
Data collection method: Observational + food frequency questionnaire
Sample type: Opportunistic
Sample size: 40
Response rate: NK
Date study carried out: NK

Comments
Sample of 40 subjects, mixed genders (20 male, 20 female), median age 4.0 years, mother completed the FFQ. Children tested individually with control and 'taste' condition and novel foods

---

Persson *et al.* (1985)
Sweden

Purpose
Descriptive

Design
Study type: Longitudinal study
Data type: Quantitative
Data collection method: Interview – closed when infant 1 year, dental examination at 3 years
Sample type:
Sample size: 312
Response rate:
Date study carried out: 1979, 1982/3

Peterson *et al.* (1984)
Montana, US

Purpose
Explanatory

Design
Study type: Experimental
Data type: Quantitative
Data collection method: Questionnaires (inc. the BET) and observation
Sample type: Random
Sample size: 106 children
Response rate: NK
Date study carried out: NK

Comments
Sample 5- and 6-year-olds
3 control classes ($n = 50$)

3 experimental ($n = 56$)
mixed genders

Pill and Parry (1989)
South Wales

Purpose
Descriptive

Design
Study type: Longitudinal
Data type: Qualitative
Data collection method: Semi-structured interviews + focus groups
Sample type: Purposive
Sample size: 130
Response rate: 65%
Date study carried out: NK

Reed (1996)
US

Purpose
Descriptive

Design
Study type: Cross-sectional
Data type: Qualitative
Data collection method: Focus group
Sample type: Opportunistic
Sample size: 20 mothers
Response rate: NK
Date study carried out: NK

Reiff and Essock-Vitale (1985)
Los Angeles, US

Purpose
Descriptive

Design
Study type: Cross-sectional
Data type: Quantitative
Data collection method: Staff-questionnaire, structured interview with mothers + medical records
Sample type: Total sample staff, opportunistic sampling with mothers
Sample size: 50 staff, 77 mothers
Response rate: 91% staff, 85% mothers
Date study carried out: 1983

Retallack *et al.* (1994)
Adelaide, Australia

Purpose
Descriptive

Design
Study type: Cross-sectional
Data type: Quantitative
Data collection method: Structured questionnaire
Sample type: Opportunistic
Sample size: 258 mothers
Response rate: 82%
Date study carried out: May–June 1992

Comments
19% of mothers did not fulfil inclusion criteria of having infant less than 53 weeks, singleton, gestational age 37 weeks or more, birth weight 2500 grams or more, no medical problems

---

Rozin *et al.* (1986)
Pennsylvania, US

Purpose
Explanatory

Design
Study type: Experimental
Data type: Quantitative
Data collection method: Observational
Sample type: Opportunistic
Sample size: 54
Response rate: NK
Date study carried out: NK

Comments
Sample of children, mean age 36.1 months, offered over 30 items of things to eat

---

Salt *et al.* (1994)
Salisbury and Durham, England

Purpose
Descriptive

Design
Study type: Cross-sectional
Data type: Quantitative
Data collection method: Questionnaire
Sample type: Quota
Sample size: 326
Response rate: 63% Salisbury
67% Durham
Date study carried out: October 1988–February 1989

Comments
In Salisbury 7% refused to take part and 29% were not in when the interviewer went to their house 5–7 weeks post-partum and in Durham 6% refused and 27% were not in

---

Santos and Booth (1996)
Birmingham, England

Purpose
Descriptive

Design
Study type: Cross-sectional
Data type: Quantitative and qualitative
Data collection method: Questionnaires and interviews – open-ended
Sample type: Opportunistic
Sample size: 158 questionnaire study, 41 interviewed
Response rate: NK
Date study carried out: October 1993

Comments
Population of students
41 students interviewed were female

Schofield, Wheeler and Stewart (1987)
London and Edinburgh, Scotland

Purpose
Descriptive

Design
Study type: Longitudinal study
Data type: Qualitative and quantitative
Data collection method: Structured interview and weighed dietary inventory and estimated food record (food diary)
Sample type: Quota
Sample size: 265 women
138 in England
127 in Scotland
Response rate: NK
Date study carried out: April 1983 to June 1985

Comments
Women visited 3 times, 8–28 weeks antenatally, 32–40 weeks, 2 months postpartum.
Women kept a weighed dietary inventory for 3 days in the third trimester.
Quota sampling to match for social class and age

Schofield, Wheeler and Stewart (1988)
London and Edinburgh, Scotland

Purpose
Descriptive

Design
Study type: Longitudinal study
Data type: Qualitative and quantitative
Data collection method: Structured interview and weighed dietary inventory and estimated food record (food diary)
Sample type: Quota
Sample size: 256 women
138 in England
127 in Scotland
Response rate: NK
Date study carried out: April 1983 to June 1985

Comments
Women visited 3 times, 8–28 weeks antenatally, 32–40 weeks, 2 months postpartum.
Women kept a weighed dietary inventory for 3 days in the third trimester.
Quota sampling to match for social class and age

Schofield, Stewart and Wheeler (1989)
London and Edinburgh, Scotland

Purpose
Descriptive

Design
Study type: Longitudinal study
Data type: Qualitative and quantitative
Data collection method: Structured interview and weighed dietary inventory and estimated food record (food diary)
Sample type: Quota
Sample size: 256 women
138 in England
127 in Scotland
Response rate: NK
Date study carried out: April 1983 to June 1985

Comments
Women visited 3 times, 8–28 weeks antenatally, 32–40 weeks, 2 months postpartum.
Women kept a weighed dietary inventory for 3 days in the third trimester.
Quota sampling to match for social class and age

Seagren and Terry (1991)
Iowa, US

Purpose
Descriptive

Design
Study type: Cross-sectional
Data type: Quantitative
Data collection method: Questionnaires, structured
Sample type: Opportunistic
Sample size: 178 female parents
Response rate: 75%
Date study carried out: 1987?

Comments
All parents were enrolled in four Iowa WIC programmes; questionnaires were completed by predominantly white parents of 130 normal weight and 48 obese children aged 3 and 4 years

---

Serdula *et al.* (1995)
16 US states

Purpose
Descriptive

Design
Study type: Cross-sectional
Data type: Quantitative
Data collection method: Telephone interviews
Sample type: Random digit

Sample size: 23699
Response rate: 'Median co-operation rate 80%'
Date study carried out: January–June 1990

Comments
Study used the Behavioural Risk Factor Surveillance System, using a FFQ composed of 6-item fruit and vegetable questionnaire developed by CDC and collected by state health department;
only adults with telephones and 'black' or 'white' included, other racial groups excluded

---

Sooman, Macintyre and Anderson (1993)
West of Scotland

Purpose
Descriptive

Design
Study type: Cross-sectional
Data type: Quantitative
Data collection method: Survey of food prices
Sample type: Shops chosen as representative on various criteria
Sample size: 10 shops per locality
Response rate: NK
Date study carried out: 1992

Comments
Survey part of West of Scotland Twenty-07 Study: Health in the Community.
Two contrasting localities chosen, with shops selected as representing various types of shop, socio-residential characteristics and geographical spread within each locality

---

Stewart, Wheeler and Schofield (1988)
England and Scotland

Purpose
Descriptive

Design
Study type: Longitudinal study
Data type: Qualitative and quantitative
Data collection method: Structured interview and weighed dietary inventory and estimated food record (food diary)
Sample type: Quota
Sample size: 256 women
138 in England
127 in Scotland
Response rate: NK
Date study carried out: April 1983 to June 1985

Comments
Women visited 3 times, 8–28 weeks antenatally, 32–40 weeks, 2 months postpartum.
Women kept a weighed dietary inventory for 3 days in the third trimester.
Quota sampling to match for social class and age

Stordy, Redfern and Morgan (1995)
5 areas of England

Purpose
Descriptive

Design
Study type: Cross-sectional
Data type: Quantitative
Data collection method: Food samples
Sample type: Purposive sample of mothers
Sample size: 265 food samples
Response rate: NK
Date study carried out: June–October 1992

Comments
Sub-sampling method not specified
Food samples from 1 meal (could be two dishes), taken away and analysed

---

Story and Resnick (1986)
Minnesota, US

Purpose
Descriptive

Design
Study type: Cross-sectional
Data type: Qualitative
Data collection method: Focus groups
Sample type: Opportunistic
Sample size: 'More than' 900 high school students
Response rate: NK
Date study carried out: NK

Comments
Part of Minnesota youth poll, uses discussion groups, 180 discussion groups of 4 to 7 people.
Exact sample size not reported

Strychar, Griffiths and Corry (1990)
British Columbia, Canada

Purpose
Descriptive

Design
Study type: Cross-sectional
Data type: Quantitative and qualitative
Data collection method: Interview
Sample type: Proportional sample
Sample size: 119
Response rate: NK
Date study carried out: June–October 1986

Comments
Interviews within 1–6 days of giving birth with primagravid women

System Three for HEBS (1994)
Scotland

Purpose
Descriptive

Design
Study type: Cross-sectional
Data type: Quantitative
Data collection method: Questionnaire
Sample type: Quota sample
Sample size: 1052 adults
Response rate: NK
Date study carried out: February–March 1994

Taras *et al.* (1989)
San Diego, US

Purpose
Descriptive

Design
Study type: Cross-sectional
Data type: Quantitative
Data collection method: Interviewer administered questionnaire
Sample type: Opportunistic
Sample size: 66 mothers
Response rate:
Date study carried out:

Comments
Children sampled from 2 age groups,
3–5 years (55%)
6–8 years (45%)

Taras and Gage (1995)
National, US

Purpose
Descriptive

Design
Study type: Content analysis
Data type: Quantitative
Data collection method: Observation
Sample type:
Sample size:
Response rate:
Date study carried out: 1993

Comments
Programmes directed at children 3.00pm–6.00pm on weekdays on 4 TV channels and Saturday am programmes on 3 major networks

Taylor and Kiblinski (1994)
Baltimore, Maryland, US

Purpose
Descriptive

Design
Study type: Cross-sectional
Data type: Quantitative
Data collection method: 24-hour dietary recall and interview
Sample type: Opportunistic
Sample size: 73 homeless mothers
Response rate: NK
Date study carried out: July 1989–March 1990

Comments
Sample includes 35 mothers and children in emergency shelters and 38 in transitional housing

Trygg *et al.* (1995)
Norway

Purpose
Descriptive

Design
Study type: Cross-sectional
Data type: Quantitative
Data collection method: Diary study, dietary records questionnaire
Sample type: Opportunistic
Sample size: 923 women
Response rate: 88% of eligible group
Date study carried out: NK

Comments
2 x 3 day dietary records on 17th and 33rd week of pregnancy

Voss, Finnis and Manners (1993)
Salisbury Health District, England

Purpose
Descriptive

Design
Study type: Cross-sectional
Data type: Quantitative
Data collection method: Postal questionnaire
Sample type: Opportunistic
Sample size: 81
Response rate: 72%
Date study carried out: May–June 1991

Wagner and Winnett (1988)
Virginia, USA

Purpose
Explanatory

Design
Study type: Experimental
Data type: Quantitative
Data collection method: Sales figures
Sample type: NK
Sample size: NK
Response rate: NK
Date study carried out: NK

Comments
2 sites used with different designs on each site.
Analysis based on sales figures

Walker (1995)
Oxford, England

Purpose
Descriptive

Design
Study type: Cross-sectional
Data type: Quantitative
Data collection method: Postal questionnaire, semi-structured
Sample type: Random
Sample size: 76
Response rate: 85%
Date study carried out: 1992

Warde and Hetherington (1994)
Greater Manchester, England

Purpose
Descriptive

Design
Study type: Cross-sectional
Data type: Quantitative
Data collection method: Questionnaire
Sample type: NK
Sample size: 323 households
Response rate: NK
Date study carried out: October/November 1990

Comments
62% of sample female
86% couples living as married
90% respondents aged between 36–55
43% of principal adult women in full-time employment

Warnke and Albrecht (1994)
US

Purpose
Descriptive

Design
Study type: Content analysis
Data type: Quantitative
Data collection method: Observation
Sample type:
Response rate:
Date study carried out: Sept, Nov 1991, January 1992

Comments
Content analysis of 3 major TV networks, Saturday am programmes and commercials viewed every third Saturday during 3-month time period.
Food mentioned or shown 11033 times

Waterson and Murray-Lyon (1989)
London, England

Purpose
Descriptive

Design
Study type: Cross-sectional
Data type: Quantitative
Data collection method: Self-completed questionnaires at 16 weeks and 28 weeks antenatally + postpartum
Sample type: Opportunistic
Sample size: 2266
Response rate: 77% (16 weeks), 51% (28 weeks)
52% (postpartum)
Date study carried out: May 1982–December 1983

Weile *et al.* (1990)
Denmark

Purpose
Descriptive

Design
Study type: Longitudinal
Data type: Quantitative
Data collection method: Interview – closed postpartum + postal questionnaires
Sample type: Opportunistic
Sample size: 500
Response rate: 500/549
Date study carried out: NK

Comments
Postal questionnaires sent to mothers at monthly intervals with 73% response rate over the year
Infants enrolled if they were less than 2000 g, gestational age of less than 36 weeks and no evidence of serious birth or underlying defects

---

Welsh Consumer Council (1993)
Wales

Purpose
Descriptive

Design
Study type: Cross-sectional
Data type: Quantitative

Data collection method: Questionnaire – shopping basket survey
Sample type: Quota
Sample size: 111
Response rate: 144 (77%)
Date study carried out: September 1988

Comments
Sectional criteria of shops: survey areas representative of Wales, urban and rural areas included, an adequate number of shops to be surveyed

---

Wheeler, Stewart and Schofield (1989)
Scotland and England

Purpose
Descriptive

Design
Study type: Longitudinal study
Data type: Qualitative and quantitative
Data collection method: Structured interview and weighed dietary inventory and estimated food record (food diary)
Sample type: Quota
Sample size: 256 women
138 in England127 in Scotland
Response rate: NK
Date study carried out: April 1983 to June 1985

Comments
Women visited 3 times, 8–28 weeks antenatally, 32–40 weeks, 2 months postpartum.
Women kept a weighed dietary inventory for 3 days in the third trimester.
Quota sampling to match for social class and age

Whichelow, Erzinclioglu and Cox (1991)
UK

Purpose
Descriptive

Design
Study type: Cross-sectional
Data type: Quantitative
Data collection method: Questionnaires
Sample type: Nationally representative
Sample size: 9003
Response rate: 73.5%
Date study carried out: 1984–1985

Comments
Data from Health and Lifestyle Survey

Winett *et al.* (1991)
Virginia, US

Purpose
Explanatory

Design
Study type: Experimental
Data type: Quantitative
Data collection method: Touchscreens
Sample type: Opportunistic then randomisation
Sample size: 61
Response rate: 61/108
Date study carried out: 1988–1989

Comments
Participants recruited over a 10-hour period, eligible if they did one large shopping per week at project supermarket. Household had two or more members and no one ate a medically prescribed diet. Baseline, intervention and follow-up

---

Winikoff *et al.* (1987)
New York, US

Purpose
Explanatory

Design
Study type: Before-and-after
Data type: Quantitative
Data collection method: Infants' medical records observation, postpartum interviews – closed with mothers, staff questionnaire
Sample type: Opportunistic
Sample size: 812 chart reviews, 16 staff + mothers (see under Comments)
Response rate: NK
Date study carried out: 1982–1985

Comments
2-year intervention following base-line study.
Interventions include staff training, breastfeeding nurse, educational materials, in-service training (staff), telephone hot-line (mothers)
Comparative study across 2 sites
sample sizes (mothers):

site 1		site 2 (control)	
1983	1985	1983	1985
60	60	148	132

Wright, Rice and Wells (1996)
Tuscon, Arizona, US

Purpose
Explanatory

Design
Study type: Before-and-after
Data type: Quantitative
Data collection method: Interviews – closed
Sample type: Opportunistic
Sample size: 192 (1990), 392 (1993)
Response rate: NK
Date study carried out: 1990–1993

Wright and Walker (1983)
Leeds, England

Purpose
Descriptive

Design
Study type: Longitudinal
Data type: Quantitative
Data collection method: Standard interview schedule
Sample type: Random
Sample size: 534
Response rate: 534/617
Date study carried out:

Comments
Random sample of first-time mothers notified to health authority. Interviews held close to 4 weeks after birth. Breastfeeding mothers re-interviewed at 4 months and 6.5 months

Wylie and Verber (1994)
UK

Purpose
Descriptive

Design
Study type: Cross-sectional
Data type: Quantitative
Data collection method: Questionnaire at booking-in + case notes + questionnaire at 4 weeks postpartum
Sample type: Opportunistic
Sample size: 576
Response rate: 96%
Date study carried out: NK

Comments
Mothers sampled from antenatal clinic

Wynn *et al.* (1994)
London, England

Purpose
Descriptive

Design
Study type: Prospective cohort
Data type: Quantitative
Data collection method: Mothers interviewed at booking visit, plus 7-day food diary completed at not more than 12 weeks antenatally
Sample type: Opportunistic
Sample size: 513
Response rate: 'About' 80%
Date study carried out:

Comments
Mothers seen as not very literate or with poor command of English not recruited

Appendix B. Surveys relevant to this review

Our knowledge of the nutritional habits of women and children in the UK is enhanced by a number of national government dietary surveys which relate specifically to the groups reviewed in this review. A number of Department of Health reports have been referred to in this review as being relevant to the age groups under study.

Women of childbearing age and pregnant women. Three surveys with nationally representative samples are relevant to this age group. Data on food consumption patterns of adults are presented in the *National Food Survey (NFS)* (MAFF). This survey reports on the amounts, costs and nutrient content of food obtained by private households in Britain. The survey includes a nationally representative sample of about 8000 households and is carried out annually. Data include a seven-day record from the householder of the description, quantity and cost of all food entering the home for human consumption. Since 1992 information about food and drink purchased outside the home, and confectionery, alcoholic and soft drinks brought into the home has been collected. Some data are analysed by gender.

The Dietary and Nutritional Survey of British Adults (Gregory *et al.*, 1990) was commissioned jointly by the Department of Health and MAFF, and carried out between October 1986 and August 1987 to collect dietary and nutritional status information on adults between the age of 16 and 64 (but excluding pregnant women). The sample size was 2197 adults living in private households in Britain. Data included a weighed food record of all food and drink consumed over seven consecutive days, and anthropometric measures (height, weight and blood pressure) and blood and urine samples. Details of social characteristics were also collected.

The Survey of Dietary Habits of 15- to 25-year-olds in Britain (Bull, 1985) took place in March to June 1982, and collected data from 452 men and 461 women aged between 15 and 25 years. Data included two-week dietary diaries to collect quantitative information about all food and drink consumed, and anthropometric (height, weight) and socioeconomic data were also collected.

The COMA report, *Dietary reference values for food energy and nutrients for the United Kingdom* (Department of Health, 1991), provides recommendations about dietary intake for adults.

Infants under the age of 1 year. There are two dietary surveys which are relevant to this age group. The OPCS (Office of Population Censuses and Surveys) carried out a series of four surveys on infant feeding patterns within the UK starting in 1975 (and covering only England and

Wales) (Martin, 1978). The next two surveys, in 1980 and 1985, covered Scotland as well (Martin and Monk, 1982; Martin and White, 1988), while the most recent one also included Northern Ireland, although the 1992 publication (White, Freeth and O'Brien, 1992) deals mainly with England, Wales and Scotland. The sample of 5413 mothers was designed to be representative of births occurring in 1990 in these four countries.

The second dietary survey, *The food and nutrient intakes of British infants aged 6–12 months* (Mills and Tyler, 1992), was commissioned by MAFF to ascertain food and nutrient intakes of older infants in Britain and to determine variation by region, socioeconomic groups and presence of other children in the family. Data include a seven-day record in which all food and drink items were specified by common household measures and recorded in a diary, followed by an interview with a parent. The sample size was 488 children, 258 children from the 6- to 9-month age group and 230 from the 9- to 12-month age group. The data were collected in November 1986.

Two COMA reports, *Present day practice in infant feeding: third report* (Department of Health and Social Security, 1988) and *Weaning and the weaning diet* (Department of Health, 1994) provide recommendations about infant liquid and solid feeding and guidance about the optimal length of breastfeeding.

Children aged 1–5 years. There is one dietary survey which relates to this age group. *The National Diet and Nutrition Survey: children aged 1½–4½* (Gregory *et al.*, 1995) was commissioned by the Department of Health and MAFF to provide information about diet and nutritional status of pre-school children living in private households in Britain. The sample of 1859 children formed a nationally representative sample, with only one child participating from each household.

Appendix C. The search strategy

Further details of the search strategy are given below.

Minimum methodological criteria for inclusion

methods: clearly stated, including study population and selection of sample, response rate and non-responders recorded, data generalisable. Methods of data gathering identified, if qualitative, data collection methods identified, biases in data collection discussed.

analysis: details of analysis explicit; statistical tests appropriate and specified, if qualitative, analytic approach described and appropriate.

interpretation of findings: appropriate to data collected.

Age/pregnancy subgroups

The review naturally falls into four subgroups, women of childbearing age, pregnant women, infants under the age of 1 and those who are between the ages of 1 and 5 years. Definition of age/pregnancy criteria were as follows:

Studies relating to women of childbearing age: this was defined as between 16 and 50 (approximately); this included studies specifically relating to adolescents although the age of the adolescent was not always specified. Few studies about single women were identified and many studies did not always define their sample by age. In a few studies women in a 55-year-old cohort have been included (for example Forsyth, Macintyre and Anderson, 1994) and 15-year-old adolescents, on the assumption that their behaviour and attitudes are unlikely to change within a year.

Studies relating to pregnant women: there were no exclusions operating with the group other than those specified below.

Studies relating to infants under the age of 1: studies did not always report upon the age of the infant although the methodology did often define indirectly the child's age, for example, where the woman was contacted 6 months after the infant's birth.

Studies relating to children aged between 1–5 years: this was a difficult selection for several reasons; studies did not always define the young child's age, but usually described them in terms of 'young', 'older' children; a number of studies took a comparative sample (studies of 5- to 10-year-olds, with cohorts of 5-, 7-, and 10-year-olds); children in American and Canadian studies were usually sampled through their school grade (for example, 'grade 1 children') the age had to be correctly identified.

Studies relating to women and men: where possible 'women-only' literature was searched but some studies were included which related to women and men when they were deemed to be important (for example, when they were part of a national sample, or on a topic about which little was written, for example vegetarians).

The exclusion criteria

A two-stage exclusion process was operated.

The first exclusion process operated at the stage of searching the literature and was weighted towards excluding studies whose topic, age group, country of study fell outside the scope of this review. Selected key words and Mesh groupings were identified for each of the four topics and applied to the four subject areas. The following exclusions were operated.

- Research relating to studies *outside the defined countries*. This particular criterion immediately excluded up to seventy per cent of some initial searches, for example, eating habits of children in most countries, many studies on breastfeeding in Third World countries, nutritional concerns with women where the country was at war (for example Bosnia), with famine, etc.

- Studies published recently but reporting on *work carried out at an earlier date (including 'historical' studies*, for example on the impact of the 'Dutch Hunger Winter' on pregnancy outcome).

- *Single case studies* (for example, of a child and his/her nutritional concerns, even when it included psychological outcomes).

- *Age groups*: studies of young adolescents or women over the age of (approximately) 50 were excluded as were studies of 'school-age' children where the *age was not specified*, or 'appeared' to be relevant only to older children (age was sometimes poorly specified).

- Studies relating to *clinical illness* (for example, low-birth-weight infant and nutritional problems, nutritional problems of sick children) or *psychological morbidity* (mothers/adolescents with eating problems, depressed women, autistic children), or *both* (chronic and severe eating problems with small children) even when this was directly relevant to nutritional factors.

- Articles reporting *social comment, author's views, political commentary, or the secondary reporting on major studies* (for example, the OPCS survey on breastfeeding published in 1990).

The second exclusion criteria operated at the next stage, once the articles had been identified and read. At this stage the extent and quality of studies in the field were known; the methodology, rigour, and standard of each study was more apparent and the focus of the study was clear.

The following criteria were used at this stage to exclude a further set of studies:

- studies *not fulfilling the minimum methodological criteria* for inclusion.

- *intervention studies.* These are covered by the companion programme funded by the Health Education Authority (HEA) if they fulfilled the following criteria: studies based on experimental or quasi-experimental designs, which included randomised controlled trials, non-randomised studies which included controlled before-and-after and interrupted time series analysis studies. There is a considerable literature reporting upon intervention studies which do not fit the HEA criteria, namely descriptive qualitative studies and studies using less rigorous quantitative methods (for example, studies of change in adopting healthy diets, nutritional intervention programmes during pregnancy, prenatal nutritional programmes in the US, studies promoting cooking skills in the UK); it was felt that they constituted a separate literature and, with exceptions, are excluded from this review. There are a few randomised controlled trials reported in the literature relating to infant feeding.

- Studies *relating to other disciplines* where the contribution was deemed too small to include (for example, 'consumer demand for new reduced-fat foods); an analysis of 'cheese expenditures' provided an in-depth economic analysis; studies reporting on analyses of health messages in consumer magazines in the US were excluded.

- Studies concerned with *food marketing* (for example, comparing supermarket interventions), consumer acquisition of commercial and nutritional information.

- Studies relating to *eating disorders* – although some studies treated eating disorders as non-psychiatric, the majority of them have been excluded as relating to a population drawn from middle-class American college students and their generalisability was questioned.

- *Studies of women and body image*: although initially it had been identified as an important area the range and nature of the studies put the topic beyond the scope of the review.

- Studies which related very specifically to *cultures/sub-cultures other than the UK*. Although studies relating to populations outside the UK are included, not all 'non-UK' studies were seen as relevant; thus studies of changes in socioeconomic status and family and food in the

US, have been excluded as have studies of homeless women and their diet in the US (but *not* the UK).

- Studies where there were *a number of studies* using a similar methodology, those with larger samples and/or a more robust reported methodology were included (for example, 'shopping basket' surveys, studies of women on low incomes and their diets; studies of women's attitudes towards breastfeeding).

Keywords. Keywords have been identified for the four topic areas and used with Mesh groupings) with the electronic searches:

Pregnancy	*Infants*
preconception	infants
pregnancy	failure to thrive
nutrition	baby
women	attitude
attitudes	weaning
views	bottle feeding
culture	culture
eating	nutrition
nutrition	weaning
food	breastfeeding
shopping	milk
work	baby
psychological factors	mother's psychology
	persuasive communication
Children aged 1–5	*Women of childbearing age*
pre-school-age-children	healthy eating
nursery schools	health education
diet	nutrition
nutrition	knowledge
eating habits	attitudes
culture	culture
feeding practices	diet
feeding	food shopping
parenting	cooking practices
eating	poverty and income
child health	meal preparation
culture	food preferences
food	food choice
children	advertising
food preferences	the media
parental attitudes	fast food
weaning	psychology

Appendix D. Experts consulted for this review

Dr Rory Williams, Dr Helen Bush and Anne Ellaway, MRC Medical Sociology Unit, Glasgow University
Members of the Department of Human Nutrition, Glasgow University
Professor Annie Anderson, School of Management and Consumer Studies, Dundee University
Dr Kathryn Backett-Milburn, Research Unit in Health and Behavioural Change, Edinburgh University
Dr Lydia Martens, Department of Applied Social Science, Stirling University
Dr Marie Reid, Department of Nutrition, Caledonian University, Glasgow
Professor Anne Murcott, School of Education and Health Studies, South Bank University, London

References

Anderson, A (1991). Food and nutrition during pregnancy: attitudes, knowledge and practice. PhD thesis. University of Aberdeen.

Anderson, A and Hunt, K (1992). Who are the healthy eaters? Eating patterns and health promotion in the west of Scotland. *Health Education Journal* **51**:3–10.

Anderson, A S, Campbell, D and Shepherd, R (1993). Nutrition knowledge, attitude to healthier eating, and dietary intake in pregnant compared to non-pregnant women. *Journal of Human Nutrition and Dietetics* **6**:335–53.

Anderson, A, Lean, M E J, Foster, A and Marshall, D (1994a). Ripe for change: fruit and vegetables in Scotland – current patterns and potential for change. *Health Bulletin* **52**:51–64.

Anderson, A, Macintyre, S and West, P (1993). Adolescent meal patterns: grazing habits in the West of Scotland. *Health Bulletin* **51**:158–65.

Anderson, A, Macintyre, S and West, P (1994). Dietary patterns among adolescents in the West of Scotland. *British Journal of Nutrition* **71**:111–12.

Anderson, A S, Hunt, K, Ford, G and Finnigan, F (1994b). One apple a day? – fruit and vegetable intake in the West of Scotland. *Health Education Research* **9**(3):297–305.

Anderson, A, Campbell, D M and Shepherd, R (1995). The influence of dietary advice on nutrient intake during pregnancy. *British Journal of Nutrition* **73**:163–77.

Anliker, J A, Laus, M J, Samonds, K W and Beal, V A (1990). Parental messages and the nutrition awareness of preschool children. *Journal of Nutrition Education* **22**:24–9.

Auerbach, K G (1984). Employed breastfeeding mothers: problems they encounter. *Birth* **11**:17–20.

Backett, K (1990). Studying health in families: a qualitative approach. In Cunningham-Burley, S and McKeganey, N (eds). *Readings in medical sociology*. London: Routledge.

Backett, K (1992) The construction of health knowledge in middle class families. *Health Education Research* **7**:497–507.

Baisch, M J, Fox, R A and Goldberg, B D (1989). Breast-feeding attitudes and practices among adolescents. *Journal of Adolescent Health Care* **10**:41–5.

Barker, D J P (1994). *Mothers, babies and disease in later life*. London: BMJ Publishing.

Beardsworth, A and Keil, T (1991). Health-related beliefs and dietary practices among vegetarians and vegans: a qualitative study. *Health Education Journal* **50**(1):38–43.

Beardsworth, A and Keil, T (1993). Contemporary vegetarianism in the UK: challenge or incorporation? *Appetite* **20**(3):229–34.

Becker, G E (1992). Breast-feeding knowledge of hospital staff in rural maternity units in Ireland. *Journal of Human Lactation* **8**:137–42.

Beeken, S and Waterston, T (1992). Health service support of breastfeeding – are we practising what we preach? *British Medical Journal* **305**:285–7.

Bergevin, Y, Dougherty, C and Kramer, M S (1983). Do infant formula samples shorten the duration of breast-feeding? *Lancet* i(8334)1148–51.

Bergman, V, Larrson, S, Lomberg, H, Marild, S and Moller, A (1994). Involvement of maternity and health care staff in breastfeeding. *Scandinavian Journal of Caring Sciences* **8**:75–80.

Best, A, Little, J and MacPherson, M (1989). Vitamin supplementation in pregnancy. *Journal of Social Health* **109**:60–3.

Birch, L L and Marlin, D W (1982). I don't like it; I never tried it: effects of exposure on two-year-old children's food preferences. *Appetite* **3**:353–60.

Birch, L L, Marlin, D and Rotter, J (1984). Eating as the 'means' activity in a contingency. *Child Development* **55**:431–9.

Birch, L L, McPhee, L, Shoba, B C, Pirok, E and Steinberg, L (1987). What kind of exposure reduces children's food neophobia: looking v. tasting. *Appetite* **9**:171–8.

Birch, L L, Johnson, S, L, Andresen, G, Peters, J and Schulte, M S (1991). The variability of young children's energy intake. *New England Journal of Medicine* **324**:232–5.

Blair, S L and Lichter, D T (1991). Measuring the division of household labor: gender segregation of housework among American couples. *Journal of Family Issues* **12**(1):91–113.

Blaxter, M (1990). *Health and Lifestyle*. London: Tavistock/Routledge.

Bloom, K, Goldbloom, R B, Robinson, S C and Stevens, F E (1982). Factors affecting the continuance of breast feeding. *Acta Paediatrica Scandinavica* (Supplement 300): 9–14.

Bruce, N G, Khan, Z and Olsen, N D L (1991). Hospital and other influences on the uptake and maintenance of breastfeeding; the development of infant feeding policy in a district. *Public Health* **105**:357–68.

Bruce, N and Griffioen, A (1995). Usefulness of a non-experimental study in the evaluation of service developments for infant feeding in a general hospital. *Social Science and Medicine* **40**:1109–16.

Bull, N (1985). Dietary habits of 15–25 year olds. *Human Nutrition* **39A** (Suppl. 1):1–68.

Cade, J and Booth, S (1990). What can people eat to meet the dietary goals: and how much does this cost? *Journal of Human Nutrition and Dietetics* **3**:199–207.

Calnan, M (1990). Food and health: a comparison of beliefs and practices in middle-class and working-class households. In Cunningham-Burley, S and McKeganey, N (eds). *Readings in Medical Sociology*. London: Routledge.

Campbell, H and Jones, I (1996). Promoting breastfeeding: a view of the current position and a proposed agenda for action in Scotland. *Journal of Public Health Medicine* **18**(4):406–14.

Campbell, H, Gorman, D and Wigglesworth, A (1995). Audit of the support for breastfeeding mothers in Fife maternity hospitals using adapted 'Baby Friendly Hospitals' materials. *Journal of Public Health Medicine* **17**(4):450–4.

Carty, E M and Bradley, C F (1990). A randomised controlled evaluation of early postpartum hospital discharge. *Birth* **17**(4):199–204.

Casey, R and Rozin, P (1989). Changing children's food preferences: parent opinions. *Appetite* **12**:171–82.

Cefalo, R C, Bowes, W A and Moos, M K (1995). Preconception care: a means of prevention. *Bailliere's Clinical Obstetrics and Gynaecology* **9**:403–16.

Central Statistical Office (1994). *Social Trends* 24.

Central Statistical Office (1995). *Social Trends* 25 .

Chalmers, J (1991). Variations in breastfeeding advice: a telephone survey of community midwives and health visitors. *Midwifery* **7**:162–6.

Chalmers, I, Enkin, M and Keirse, M J N C (1989). *Effective care in pregnancy and childbirth*. Oxford: Oxford University Press.

Charles, N and Kerr, M (1988). *Women, food and families*. Manchester: Manchester University Press.

Clark, N A C and Fisk, N M (1994). Minimal compliance with the Department of Health recommendations for routine folate prophylaxis to prevent neural tube defects. *British Journal of Obstetrics and Gynaecology* **101**(8):709–10.

Cornelius, L J (1991). Health habits of school age children. *Journal of Healthcare for the Poor and Underserved* **2**:374–85.

Cotunga, N, Subar, A F, Heimendinger, J and Kahle, L (1992). Nutrition and cancer prevention knowledge, beliefs, attitudes, and practices: the 1987 National Health Interview Survey. *Journal of the American Dietetic Association* **92**:963–8.

Cox, B, Blaxter, M, Buckle, A L J, Fenner, N P, Golding, J F, Gore, M, Huppert, F A, Nickson, J *et al.* (1987). *The Health and Lifestyle Survey: preliminary report*. London: Health Promotion Trust.

Cox, D N, Anderson, A S, McKellar, S, Reynolds, J, Lean, M E J and Mela, D J (1996). Vegetables and fruit: barriers and opportunities for greater consumption. *Nutrition and Food Science* **5**:44–7.

Cox, M, Whittle, M J, Bryne, A, Kingdom, J C P and Ryan, G (1992). Pre-pregnancy counselling: experience from 1075 cases. *British Journal of Obstetrics and Gynaecology* **99**:873–6.

Cresswell, J, Busby, A, Young, H and Inglis, V (1983). Dietary patterns of third-year secondary schoolgirls in Glasgow. *Applied Nutrition* **307A**:301–6.

Crotty, P A, Rutishauser, I H E and Cahill, M (1992). Food in low-income families. *Australian Journal of Public Health* **16**:168–74.

Davis, C N (1928). Self selection of diet by newly weaned infants: an experimental study. *American Journal of Diseases in Childhood* **36**:651–79.

Dawson, B L, Jeffrey, D B and Walsh, J A (1988). Televised food commercials' effect on children's resistance to temptation. *Journal of Applied Social Psychology* **18**:1353–60.

Department for Education and Employment (1996). *Education statistics for the United Kingdom: 1995 edition*. London: HMSO.

Department of Health and Social Security (1984). *Diet and Cardiovascular Disease*. Report of the Committee on Medical Aspects of Food Policy. Report on Health and Social Subjects No. 28. London: HMSO.

Department of Health and Social Security (1988). *Present day practice in infant feeding: third report*. Report on Health and Social Subjects No. 32. London: HMSO.

Department of Health (1991). *Dietary reference values for food energy and nutrients for the United Kingdom*. Report on Health and Social Subjects No. 41. London: HMSO.

Department of Health (1992). *The health of the nation: a strategy for health in England*. London: HMSO.

Department of Health (1994). *Weaning and the weaning diet*. Report on Health and Social Subjects No. 45. London: HMSO.

Devine, C and Olson, C M (1992). Women's perceptions about the way social roles promote or constrain personal nutrition care. *Women and Health* **19**:79–95.

Dittus, K L, Hillers, V N and Beerman, K A (1995). Benefits and barriers to fruit and vegetable intake: relationship between attitudes and consumption. *Journal of Nutrition Education* **27**(3):120–6.

Dobson, B, Beardsworth, T, Keil, T and Walker, R (1994). *Diet, choice and poverty: social, cultural and nutritional aspects of food consumption among low-income families.* Loughborough: Loughborough University of Technology Centre for Research in Social Policy.

Douthitt, R A (1989). The division of labor within the home: have gender roles changed? *Sex Roles* **20**(11–12):693–704.

Dowler, E and Calvert, C (1995). *Nutrition and diet in lone-parent families in London.* London: Family Policy Studies Centre.

Doyal, L (1995). *What makes women sick? Gender and the political economy of health.* Basingstoke: Macmillan.

Doyle, W, Crawford, M A, Laurance, B M and Drury, P (1982). Dietary survey during pregnancy in socioeconomic groups. *Human Nutrition: Applied Nutrition* **36A**:95–106.

Drake, M A (1992). The nutritional status and dietary adequacy of single homeless women and their children in shelters. *Public Health Reports* **107**(3):312–18.

Dusdieker, L B, Booth, B M, Seals, B F and Ekwo, E E (1985). Investigation of a model for the initiation of breastfeeding in primagravida women. *Social Science and Medicine* **20**:695–703.

Eiser, C and Eiser, J R (1985). Health education of the primigravidae. *Child: Care, Health and Development* **11**:53–60.

Ellis, D J (1983). Secondary school students' attitudes and beliefs about breastfeeding. *Journal of School Health* **53**:600–4.

Evans, C J, Lyons, N B and Killien, M G (1986). The effect of infant formula samples on breastfeeding practice. *Journal of Obstetric Gynecologic and Neonatal Nursing* **15**:401–5.

Expert Advisory Group (1992). *Folic acid and the prevention of neural tube defects.* London: Department of Health.

Fantasia, R (1995). Fast-food in France. *Theory and Society* **24**(2):201–43.

Forsyth, A, Macintyre, S and Anderson, A (1994). Diets for disease? Intra-urban variation in reported food consumption in Glasgow. *Appetite* **22**:259–74.

Frank, D A, Wirtz, S J, Sorenson, J R and Heeren, T (1987). Commercial discharge packs and breastfeeding counselling: effects on infant-feeding practices in a randomized trial. *Pediatrics* **80**:845–54.

Freed, G L and Fraley, J K (1993). Effect of expectant mothers' feeding plan on prediction of fathers' attitudes regarding breast-feeding. *American Journal of Perinatology* **10**(4):300–3.

Fuller, S and Mackie, I (1996). Marketing baby foods through the NHS: mothers' views. *Health Visitor* **69**(9):363–4.

Furst, T, Connors, M, Bisogni, C, Sobal, J and Falk, L W (1996). Food choice: a conceptual model of the process. *Appetite* **26**:247–66.

Gabriel, A, Gabriel, K R and Lawrence, R A (1986). Cultural values and biomedical knowledge: choices in infant feeding. Analysis of a survey. *Social Science and Medicine* **23**(5):501–9.

Galst, J and White, M (1976). The unhealthy persuader: the reinforcing value of television and children's purchasing-influencing attempts at the supermarket. *Child Development* **47**:1089–96.

Gibney, M J and Lee, P (1993). Patterns of food and nutrient intake in a suburb of Dublin with chronically high unemployment. *Journal of Human Nutrition and Dietetics* **6**:13–22.

Goodine, L A and Fried, P A (1984). Infant feeding practices: pre- and postnatal factors affecting choice and method and the duration of breastfeeding. *Canadian Journal of Public Health* **75**:439–44.

Gorn, G J and Goldberg, M E (1982). Behavioural evidence of the effects of televised food messages on children. *Journal of Consumer Research* **9**(2):200–5.

Graham, H (1984). *Women, health and the family.* London: Harvester Press.

Graham, H (1993). *Hardship and health in women's lives.* London: Harvester Wheatsheaf.

Gregg, J E M (1989). Attitudes of teenagers in Liverpool to breastfeeding. *British Medical Journal* **299**:148–9.

Gregory, J, Foster, K, Tyler, H and Wiseman, M (1990). *Dietary and nutritional survey of British adults.* London: HMSO.

Gregory, J, Collins, D L, Davies, P S W, Hughes, J and Clarke, P C (1995). *National diet and nutrition: children aged one-and-a-half to four-and-a-half years.* London: HMSO.

Grossman, L K, Fitzsimmons, S M, Larsen-Alexander, J B, Sachs, L and Harter, C (1990). The infant feeding decision in low and upper income women. *Clinical Pediatrics* **29**(1):30–7.

Hally, M R, Bond, J, Crawley, J, Gregson, B, Philips, P and Russell, I (1984). Factors influencing the feeding of first-born infants. *Acta Paediatrica Scandinavica* **73**:33–9.

Hamilton, M B (1993). Wholefoods and health foods: beliefs and attitudes. *Appetite* **20**(3):223–8.

Haste, F M, Brooke, O G, Anderson, H R, Bland, J M, Shaw, A, Griffin, J and Peacock, J L (1990). Nutrient intakes during pregnancy: observations on the influence of smoking and social class. *American Journal of Clinical Nutrition* **51**:29–36.

Heald, F P and Felix, P (1992). Fast food and snack food: beneficial or deleterious. *Journal of Adolescent Health* **13**:380–3.

Health Education Authority (1989). *Diet, nutrition and 'healthy eating' in low income groups.* London: Health Education Authority.

Hill, G M (1995). The impact of breakfast especially ready-to-eat cereals on nutrient intake and health of children. *Nutrition Research* **15**:595–613.

Holt, G M and Wolkind, S N (1983). Early abandonment of breast feeding: causes and effects. *Child: Care, Health and Development* **9**(6):349–55.

James, A (1979). Confections, concoctions and conceptions. *Journal of the Anthropological Society of Oxford* **10**(2):83.

James, D (1981). Breast feeding in Manchester. *Public Health* **95**:334–43.

Jeffrey, D B, McLellarn, R W and Fox, D T (1982). The development of children's eating habits: the role of television commercials. *Health Education Quarterly* **9**(2–3):174–89.

Jensen, T D, Rao, C P and Hilton, R (1989). Working versus nonworking wives' psychographic profiles: a longitudinal analysis. *Journal of Business Research* **19**(4)255–66.

Johnson, R K, Smiciklas-Wright, H and Crouter, A C (1992). Effect of maternal employment on the quality of young children's diets: the CSFII experience. *Journal of the American Dietetic Association* **92**:213–14.

Jones, D A (1987). The choice to breast feed or bottle feed and influences upon that choice: a survey of 1525 mothers. *Child: Care, Health and Development* **13**:75–85.

Jones, D A and West, R R (1986). Effect of a lactation nurse on the success of breast-feeding: a randomised controlled trial. *Journal of Epidemiology and Community Health* **40**(1):45–9.

Kilcast, D, Cathro, J and Morris, L (1996). Practical approaches to increasing vegetable consumption. *Nutrition and Food Science* **5**:48–51.

Kim, C (1989). Working wives' time-saving tendencies: durable ownership, convenience food consumption, and meal purchases. *Journal of Economic Psychology* **10**(3):391–409.

Kitzinger, S (1980). *Women as mothers.* New York: Vintage Books.

Klesges, R C, Stein, R J, Eck, L H, Isbell, T R and Klesges, L M (1991). Parental influences on food selection in young children. *American Journal of Clinical Nutrition* **53**:859–64.

Kogan, M D, Alexander, G R, Kotelchuck, M, Nagey, D A and Jack, B W (1994). Comparing mothers' reports on the content of prenatal care received with recommended national guidelines for care. *Public Health Reports* **109**:637–46.

Koivisto, U K, Fellenius, J and Sjøden, P O (1994). Relations between parental mealtime practices and children's food intake. *Appetite* **22**:245–57.

Kotz, K and Story, M (1994). Food advertisements during children's Saturday morning television programming: Are they consistent with dietary recommendations? *Journal of the American Dietetic Association* **94**:1296–300.

Lang, T and Baker, L (1993). The decline of cooking. *Modus*, October, pp. 200–2.

Laurent, C (1993). Private function? *Nursing Times* **89**(47):14–15.

Levitt, C (1993) Preconception health promotion. *Primary Care* **20**:537–49.

Lilburne, A M, Oates, R K, Thompson, S and Tong, L (1988). Infant feeding in Sydney: a survey of mothers who bottle feed. *Australian Paediatric Journal* **24**:49–54.

Lindberg, L, Bohlin, G and Hagekull, B (1994). Early food refusal: infant and family characteristics. *Infant Mental Health Journal* **15**:262–77.

Lobstein, T (1988). *Fast food facts: a survival guide to the good, the bad and the really ugly of fast foods.* London Food Commission. London: Camden Press.

London Food Commission (ed.) (undated) *Food retailing in London: a pilot study of the three largest retailers and Londoners' access to food.* CES Limited.

Low Income Project Team for the Nutrition Task Force (1996). *Low income, food, nutrition and health.* London: Department of Health.

Lucas, A (1994). Role of nutritional programming in determining adult morbidity. *Archives of Disease in Childhood* **71**:288–90.

Lumley, J and Astbury, J (1989). Advice for pregnancy. In Chalmers, I, Enkin, M and Keirse, M J N C. *Effective Care in Pregnancy and Childbirth.* Oxford: Oxford University Press.

McIntosh, J (1985). Barriers to breastfeeding: choice of feeding method in a sample of working class primiparae. *Midwifery* **1**:213–24.

McIntosh J (1986). Weaning practices in a sample of working class primiparae. *Child: Care, Health and Development* **12**:215–26.

McIntyre, L (1993). A survey of breakfast-skipping and inadequate breakfast-eating among young schoolchildren in Nova Scotia. *Canadian Journal of Public Health* **84**:410–14.

McIntyre, L and Horbul, B A (1995). A survey of breakfast-eating among young schoolchildren in Northeastern Ontario. *Canadian Journal of Public Health* **86**:305–8.

Mackie, L J, Wood, R C and Gregory, S (1993). Women defining health: food, diet and body image. *Health Education Research* **8**(1):35–41.

McKillop, F M and Durnin, J C (1982). The energy and nutrient intake of a random sample of infants. *Human Nutrition: Applied Nutrition* **36A**:405–21.

Maehr, J C, Lizarraga, J L,Wingard, D L and Felice, M E (1993). A comparative study of adolescent and adult mothers who intend to breastfeed. *Journal of Adolescent Health* **14**:453–7.

Mander, R (1995). Advertising infant formula in the maternity area. *MIDIRS Midwifery Digest* **5**(3)338–41.

Manstead, A S, Proffitt, C and Smart, J L (1983). Predicting and understanding mothers' infant-feeding intentions and behaviour: testing the theory of reasoned action. *Journal of Personality and Social Psychology* **44**(4):657–71.

Manstead, A S, Plevin, C E and Smart, J L (1984). Predicting mothers' choice of infant feeding method. *British Journal of Social Psychology* **23**(3):223–31.

Martens, L and Warde, A (1997). Urban pleasure? On the meaning of eating out in a northern city. In Caplan, P (ed.) *Food, health and identity*. London: Routledge.

Martin, J (1978). *Infant feeding 1975: attitudes and practices in England and Wales.* London: HMSO.

Martin, J and Monk, J (1982). *Infant feeding 1980.* London: Office of Population Censuses and Surveys.

Martin, J and White, A (1988). *Infant feeding 1985.* London: HMSO.

Matich, J R and Sims, L S (1992). A comparison of social support variables between women who intend to breast or bottle feed. *Social Science and Medicine* **34**(8):919–27.

Mayall, B (1986). *Keeping children healthy: the role of mothers and professionals.* London: Allen & Unwin.

Medical Research Council Vitamin Study Research Group (1991). Prevention of neural tube defects: results of the Medical Research Council Vitamin Study. *Lancet* **338**:131–7.

Mills, A and Tyler, H (1992). *Food and nutritional intakes of British infants aged 6–12 months.* London: HMSO.

Ministry of Agriculture, Fisheries and Food (1994). *National Food Survey: annual report on household food consumption and expenditure.* London: HMSO.

Ministry of Agriculture, Fisheries and Food (1995). *National Food Survey: annual report on household food consumption and expenditure.* London: HMSO.

Ministry of Agriculture, Fisheries and Food (1996). *National Food Survey: annual report on household food consumption and expenditure.* London: HMSO.

Ministry of Agriculture, Fisheries and Food (1995). *Nutritional Labelling Study.* London: HMSO.

Mooney, C (1990). Cost and availability of healthy food choices in a London health district. *Journal of Human Nutrition and Dietetics* **3**:111–20.

Morgan, J B, Kimber, A C, Redfern, A M and Stordy, B J (1995). Healthy eating for infants – mothers' attitudes. *Acta Paediatrica* **84**:512–15.

Morgan, J and Stordy, J (1995). Infant feeding practices in the 1990s. *Health Visitor* **68**(2):56–9.

Morrow, M and Barraclough, S (1993). Breast-feeding and public policy in Australia: limitations of a nutritional focus. *Health Promotion International* **8**(2):135–46.

Mulliner, C M, Spiby, H and Fraser, R B (1995). A study exploring midwives' education in, knowledge of, and attitudes to, nutrition in pregnancy. *Midwifery* **11**:37–41.

Murcott, A (1982). On the social significance of the 'cooked dinner' in South Wales. *Social Science Information* **21**(4/5):677–96.

Murcott, A (1983). It's a pleasure to cook for him: food, mealtime and gender in some South Wales households. In Garmarnikow, E, Morgan, D, Purvis, J and Taylorson, D (eds). *The public and the private.* London: Heinemann.

Murcott, A (1988). On the altered appetites of pregnancy – conceptions of food, body and person. *Sociological Review* **36**(4):733–64.

Murcott, A (1997). Family meals: a thing of the past. In Caplan, P (ed.). *Food, health and identity.* London: Routledge.

Murphy, A S, Youatt, J P, Hoerr, S L, Sawyer, C A and Andrews, S L (1995). Kindergarten students' food preferences are not consistent with their knowledge of the dietary guidelines. *Journal of the American Dietetic Association* **95**:219–23.

Murray, S, Narayan, V, Mitchell, M and Witte, H (1993). Study of dietetic knowledge among members of the primary health care team. *British Journal of General Practice* **43**:229–31.

National Children's Homes (1991). *NCH Poverty and Nutrition Survey* (1991). London: National Children's Homes.

Neifert, M, Gray, J, Gary, N and Camp, B (1988a). Effect of two types of hospital feeding gift packs on duration of breastfeeding among adolescent mothers. *Journal of Adolescent Health Care* **9**:411–13.

Neifert, M, Gray, J, Gary, N and Camp, B(1988b). Factors influencing breastfeeding among adolescents. *Journal of Adolescent Health Care* **9**:470–3.

Nolan, L, and Goel, V (1995). Socio-demographic factors related to breastfeeding in Ontario: results from the Ontario Health Survey. *Canadian Journal of Public Health* **86**(5):309–12.

Oakley, A (1980). *Women confined.* Oxford: Martin Robertson.

Oakley, A and Rajan, L (1993). What did your baby eat today? Social factors and infant feeding practices. *European Journal of Public Health* **3**:18–27.

Olson, P N, Ponzetti, J J and Olson, G I (1989). Time demands on families: is there a bottom line? *Lifestyles* **10**(4):311–23.

Parraga, I M (1990). Determinants of food consumption. *Journal of American Dietetic Association* **90**:661–3.

Payne, M and Payne, B (1993). *Eating out in the UK: market structure, consumer attitudes and prospects for the 1990s.* Special Report No. 2169. London: Economist Intelligence Unit.

Pearson, S, Dimond, H, Ford, F and Fraser, R (1996). A survey of pre-pregnancy nutritional knowledge in family planning clinics. *British Journal of Family Planning* **22**:92–4.

Pelchat, M L and Pliner, P (1995). 'Try it, you'll like it'. *Appetite* **24**:153–65.

Persson, L, Holm, A, Arvidsson, S and Samuelson, G (1985). Infant feeding and dental caries – a longitudinal study of Swedish children. *Swedish Medical Journal* **9**:201–6.

Peterson, P E, Jeffrey, D B, Bridgwater, C A and Dawson, B (1984). How pronutrition television programmes affect children's dietary habits. *Developmental Psychology* **20**:55–63.

Pill, R and Parry, O (1989). Making changes – women, food and families. *Health Education Journal* **48**:51–4.

Reed, D B (1996). Focus groups identify desirable features of nutrition programs for low-income mothers of preschool children. *Journal of the American Dietetic Association* **96**:501–3.

Rees, J M (1992). The overall impact of recently developed foods on the dietary habits of adolescents. *Journal of Adolescent Health* **13**(5):389–91.

Reid, M and Garcia, J (1989). Women's views of care during pregnancy and childbirth. In Chalmers, I, Enkin, M and Keirse, M J N C. *Effective Care in Pregnancy and Childbirth.* Oxford: Oxford University Press.

Reiff, M I and Essock-Vitale, S M (1985). Hospital influences on early infant-feeding practices. *Pediatrics* **76**:872–9.

Retallack, S J, Simmer, K, Makrides, M and Gibson, R A (1994). Infant weaning practices in Adelaide: the results of a shopping complex survey. *Journal of Paediatric Child Health* **30**:28–32.

Rozin, P, Hammer, L, Oster, H, Horowitz, T and Marmora, V (1986). The child's conception of food: differentiation of categories of rejected substances in the 16 months to 5 year age range. *Appetite* **7**:141–51.

Salt, M J, Law, C M, Bull, A R and Osmond, C (1994). Determinants of breastfeeding in Salisbury and Durham. *Journal of Public Health Medicine* **16**:291–5.

Santos, M L S and Booth, D A (1996). Influences on meat avoidance among British students. *Appetite* **27**:197–205.

Schofield, C, Wheeler, E and Stewart, J (1987). The diets of pregnant and post-pregnant women in different social groups in London and Edinburgh: energy, protein, fat and fibre. *British Journal of Nutrition* **58**:369–81.

Schofield, E C, Wheeler, E F and Stewart, J D (1988). Is the message getting through? Nutritional knowledge of pregnant women in Edinburgh and London. *European Journal of Clinical Nutrition* **42**:161–7.

Schofield, C, Stewart, J and Wheeler, E (1989). The diets of pregnant and post-pregnant women in different social groups in London and Edinburgh: calcium, iron, retinol, ascorbic acid and folic acid. *British Journal of Nutrition* **62**:363–77.

Scottish Office Home and Health Department (1993). *The Scottish diet.* Edinburgh: Scottish Office Home and Health Department.

Scottish Office (1996). *Scotland's health: a challenge to us all.* Edinburgh: Scottish Office Department of Health.

Seagren, J S and Terry, R D (1991). WIC female parents' behavior and attitudes toward their children's food intake – relationship to children's relative weight. *Journal of Nutrition Education* **23**:223–30.

Serdula, M K, Coates, R J, Byers, T, Simoes, E, Mokdad, A H and Subar, A F (1995). Fruit and vegetable intake among adults in 16 states: results of a brief telephone survey. *American Journal of Public Health* **85**:236–9.

Sooman, A, Macintyre, S and Anderson, A (1993). Scotland's health – a more difficult challenge for some? The price and availability of healthy foods in socially contrasting localities in the West of Scotland. *Health Bulletin* **51**:276–84.

Sorensen, G, Hunt, M K, Morris, D H and Donnelly, G (1990). Promoting healthy eating patterns in the worksite: the Treatwell intervention model. *Health Education Research* **5**(4):505–15.

Stewart, J, Wheeler, E and Schofield, C (1988). Regional differences in British attitudes to diet in pregnancy: priorities and pragmatism. *Ecology of Food and Nutrition* **20**:211–29.

Stitt, S, Jepson, M and Paulson-Box, E (1995). Taking the cooking out of food: nutrition and the national curriculum. *Nutrition and Health* **10**:155–64.

Stordy, B J, Redfern, A M and Morgan, J B (1995). Healthy eating for infants – mothers actions. *Acta Paediatrica* **84**:733–41.

Story, M (1989). A perspective on adolescent snacking behaviour. *National Dairy Council Nutrition News* **52**:1–3.

Story, M and Brown, J E (1987). Sounding board: do young children instinctively know what to eat? *New England Journal of Medicine* **316**:103–5.

Story, M and Resnick, M D (1986). Adolescents' views on food and nutrition. *Journal of Nutrition Education* **18**:188–92.

Strychar, I M, Griffiths, W S and Conry, R F (1990). The relationship among learning, health beliefs, alcohol consumption, and tobacco use of primigravidas. *Canadian Journal of Public Health* **81**:462–7.

System Three for HEBS (1994). *Breastfeeding*. Edinburgh: Health Education Board for Scotland.

Taras, H L, Sallis, J F, Patterson, T L, Nader, P R and Nelson, J A (1989). Television's influence on children's diet and physical activity. *Journal of Development and Pediatrics* **10**(4):176–80.

Taras, H L and Gage, M (1995). Advertised foods on children's television. *Archives of Pediatrics and Adolescent Medicine* **149**:649–52.

Taylor, M L and Kiblinsky, S A (1994). Food consumption and eating behavior of homeless preschool children. *Journal of Nutrition Education* **26**:20–5.

Trygg, K, Lund Larsen, K, Sandstad, B, Hoffman, H J, Jacobsen, G and Bakketeig, L S (1995). Do pregnant smokers eat differently from pregnant non-smokers? *Paediatric and Perinatal Epidemiology* **9**:307–19.

Turner, T (1996). Baby-friendly frenzy. *Health Visitor* **69**(9):350–1.

US Department of Health and Human Services Public Health Service (1993). 1992 National Survey of Worksite Health Promotion Activities: summary. *American Journal of Health Promotion* **7**(6):452–64.

Voss, S, Finnis, L and Manners, J (1993). Fathers and breastfeeding: a pilot observational study. *Journal of the Royal Society of Health*, August, pp. 176–8.

Wagner, J L and Winett, R A (1988). Prompting one low-fat, high-fibre selection in a fast-food restaurant. *Journal of Applied Behavior Analysis* **21**(2):179–85.

Walker, C (1995). When to wean: whose advice do mothers find helpful? *Health Visitor* **68**(3):109–11.

Warde, A and Hetherington, K (1994). English households and routine food practices: a research note. *Sociological Review* **42**:758–78.

Warnke, M R and Albrecht, J A (1994). Media portrayal of foods during Saturday morning television programming and in children's magazines. *Journal of Consumer Studies and Home Economics* **18**:85–95.

Waterson, E J and Murray-Lyon, I M (1989). Drinking and smoking patterns amongst women attending an antenatal clinic – 11. During pregnancy. *Alcohol and Alcoholism* **24**(2):163–73.

Weile, B, Rubin, D H, Krasilnikoff, P A, Kuo, H S and Jekel, J F (1990). Infant feeding patterns during the first year of life in Denmark: factors associated with the discontinuation of breast-feeding. *Journal of Clinical Epidemiology* **43**:1305–11.

Welsh Consumer Council (1993). *Shopping for food: a study of food prices and availability in Wales*. Cardiff: Welsh Consumer Council.

Wheeler, E, Stewart, J and Schofield, C (1989). Dietary variety during and after pregnancy in Scotland and England. *Journal of Human Nutrition and Dietetics* **2**:7–18.

Whichelow, M J, Erzinclioglu, S W and Cox, B D (1991). Some regional variations in dietary patterns in a random sample of British adults. *European Journal of Clinical Nutrition* **45**:253–62.

White, A, Freeth, S and O'Brien, M (1992). *Infant feeding 1990*. London: HMSO.

Winett, R A, Wagner, J L, Moore, J F and Walker, W B *et al.* (1991) An experimental evaluation of a prototype public access nutrition information system for supermarkets. *Health Psychology* **10**(1):75–8.

Winikoff, B, Laukaran, V H, Myers, D and Stone, R (1987). Dynamics of infant feeding: mothers, professionals, and the institutional context in a large urban hospital. *Pediatrics* **77**:357–65.

World Health Organization (1989). Infant feeding: the physiological basis. Bulletin **67**: supplement.

Woollett, A (1987). Who breastfeeds? The family and cultural context. *Journal of Reproductive and Infant Psychology* **5**(3):127–31.

Wright, H J and Walker, P C (1983). Prediction of duration of breast feeding in primiparas. *Journal of Epidemiology and Community Health* **37**(2):89–94.

Wright, J (1996). Breastfeeding and deprivation – the Nottingham peer counsellor programme. *MIDIRS Midwifery Digest* **6**(2):212–15.

Wright, A, Rice, S and Wells, S (1996). Changing hospital practices to increase the duration of breastfeeding. *Pediatrics* **97**(5):669–75.

Wylie, J and Verber, I (1994). Why women fail to breastfeed: a prospective study from booking to 28 days post-partum. *Journal of Human Nutrition and Dietetics* **7**:115–120.

Wynn, S W, Wynn, A H A, Doyle, W and Crawford, M A (1994). Maternal social class, maternal diet and dimensions of babies in a population of London women. *Nutrition and Health* **9**:303–15.

Young, B and Hetherington, M (1996). The literature on advertising and children's food choice. *Nutrition and Food Science* **5**:15–18.